This Book Is Certified to Be

WOSWAK* Free

Warmed-Over Stuff We Already Knew

the GREAT FAT FRAUD

Why the "Obesity Epidemic" isn't, how
to be totally healthy without losing weight
and if you should lose some pounds, how
to keep them from finding you again

Mike Schatzki

Lamington Press
Bedminster, NJ

V 1.0
Printed in the United States of America.

Information: Lamington Press
              www.LamingtonPress.com
              Info@LamingtonPress.com

Publisher's Cataloging-in-Publication Data

Schatzki, Michael.
    The great fat fraud : why the "obesity epidemic" isn't, how
to be totally healthy without losing weight and if you should
lose some pounds, how to keep them from finding you
again / Mike Schatzki.
        p. cm.
    Includes bibliographical references.
    ISBN: 978-0-9837725-4-5 (pbk.)
    ISBN: 978-0-9837725-5-2 (e-book: ePub)
    1. Weight loss—Health aspects. 2. Obesity—Health
aspects. 3. Health behavior.   I. Title.
RM222.2 .S261 2011
613.7—dc22

                                              2011934174

Contents

1

Schatzki, You Idiot

Schatzki, you idiot, what do you mean the Obesity Epidemic isn't? Everybody KNOWS there's an Obesity Epidemic. We all KNOW that fat is bad, bad, bad. We all KNOW that losing weight is good, good, good. The government says that one-third of Americans are overweight and another third are obese. People are dropping like flies from the disease of obesity.

How can you possibly say that there isn't an Obesity Epidemic?

Well, I think that Mark Twain said it best: "It ain't what you don't know that gets you into trouble. It's what you know for sure that just ain't so."

And when it comes to obesity, what everybody "knows for sure" just ain't so. So how come we believe it? Because the $58 billion Weight Loss Industry has been so fantastically successful in ignoring reality and selling us this incredible bill of goods called the "Obesity Epidemic."

> *How do I know you're right when everyone else thinks it "is just so?"*

Because I can prove it to you.

> *How?*

Let's go to the research and I will show you.

2

Research Is So Boring

RESEARCH? You have to be kidding. Research is so boring. You know, they come up with research studies like "The Effect of Duck Quacking on Hearing Aid Battery Life."

True, true. The academic publish-or-perish imperative turns out tons of papers, not all of which are earthshaking. But it also turns out some really good stuff, stuff that absolutely demolishes the Great Fat Fraud and turns conventional wisdom on its head.

Great. So I just have to trust that you, genius that you are, have laid it all out for me and I can believe everything you say.

Well actually, I believe in "trust but verify." So every time I reference a research study in the book, I'll put a endnote number by it. The endnotes are in Part VII of the book. They will have more detail about the science involved and you'll be able to see exactly which research study I'm talking about and what it says.

Wooptydo! Like I have a medical research library right down the street and can just drop in any time and grab a quick copy of the New England Journal of Medicine.

Ten years ago, that is exactly what you would've had to do. But now it's so much easier. Most of the best journals allow you to download their articles for free immediately or after a fixed period of time. And most of the key research that has been so carefully ignored has been around that long and often much longer. So not only will I give you the article citation, but also the website address so that you can go and download the article for yourself.

Well good, but I still have to type out those long web addresses, probably make a mistake and never find the article.

All you have to do is type in one website address. Go to www.greatfatfraud.com and click on the "Book Reference Links" page. Go to the article you want to read, and click on the link and that will take you right to it.

> *Okay, but those articles are really tough to read. They're all full of statistical gobbledygook and highfalutin academiceese.*

You're absolutely right. Academics and researchers don't write for us, they write for each other. They don't really expect us to read their research and they frankly don't much care, in most cases, what we think about it. Furthermore, most of them are horrendous communicators. They hide their most interesting, earthshaking discovery in line 8 of table 3, mention it briefly in their summary, and end with the obligatory plea for more research.

Therefore, if you go ahead and download a paper, the endnote for that paper will tell you exactly where to look for the key golden nuggets that the researchers have come up with and that we are going to be focusing on.

PART
I

How To Be Totally Healthy

without Losing a Pound

3

Fitlessness

Many studies will tell you that if you look at the total population, being heavy results in really bad things, such as dramatically increasing your risk of dying.[1]

But it's not about weight at all. Weight can make things worse, but if you fix the underlying cause, what you weigh becomes irrelevant!

What is it that you have to fix? Well, first we need a little background for this all to make sense.

It has long been suspected that people afflicted with Fitlessness had a higher death rate from cardiovascular and other diseases. Believe it or not, someone actually did a study in 1864 showing that tailors, who mostly sat all day, had a much higher mortality rate than agricultural workers.[2]

However, the first really modern quantitative epidemiological study on the impact of Fitlessness on mortality rates was published by Dr. Jeremy Morris in 1953.[3] He studied drivers and conductors on English double-decker buses and discovered that the conductors, who climbed up and down the steps many times a day, had a 50 percent reduction in their chance of dying of a heart attack compared to the relatively inactive drivers who sat most of the day.

In order to make sure that this wasn't caused by the nature of the conductors' interaction with passengers, he also studied...

*Wait a minute. **WAIT A MINUTE!** I got it. I have so got it! Fitlessness = Not Being Fit. I CAN'T BELIEVE IT. This whole book is going to turn into a sermon on exercise? Sweat, get your heart rate up, no pain no gain. Please, spare me. I don't like exercise. I tried it once and it didn't agree with me.*

Don't Panic!

I absolutely promise you, I totally guarantee that in order to be fit enough to be really healthy and reduce your chances of dying of anything by at least 50 percent, regardless of your weight...

You Don't Need to Exercise

So give me just a page or two to layout the science of how fitness has a critical relationship to what's called all-cause mortality, that is, your chances of dying of anything.

But this is a book on weight, right? What has this fitness stuff got to with weight?

Shortly will you see and amazed will you be

So hang in there for moment and we will get there.

Anyway, to make sure that the results didn't have something to do with the conductors' interactions with passengers (he was a very careful and meticulous researcher), he repeated the study with postal workers and found that clerks and telephone operators, who had lots of customer contact, had twice the cardiac mortality rate of postal workers who delivered the mail on foot or by bike. Thus, he concluded that physical activity provided protection against cardiac arrest.

In the more than fifty years since this seminal study appeared, it has been conclusively proven that if you are reasonably fit, you can dramatically cut your chances of dying, not only from cardiac disease, but from anything (all-cause mortality). And that you can become reasonably fit without traditional exercise (that is without running, jogging, biking, swimming, aerobic dance, in-line skating, etc.).

For example, Dr. Steven Blair and colleagues published a study in 1989 that analyzed the records of 10,000 men and 3,000 women who had taken a treadmill fitness test and were then followed for eight years. The all-cause mortality rates of those participants who were reasonably fit (levels of fitness that can be achieved without exercise) were significantly lower than those who were sedentary.[4]

Similar studies published in 2002 and 2008 by Jonathan Myers and Peter Kokkinos, looking at a different population of individuals who had also taken treadmill fitness tests, found similar results.[5,6]

The bottom line is that the scientists and researchers have conclusively proven that achieving a level of fitness that can be obtained without exercise will cut your chances of dying of anything by at least 50 percent. This is now accepted as part of the basic laws of human biology and physiology.

Okay, what does all this have to do with weight? Well, this is where it really gets interesting.

4

Drs. Morris, Blair, Wei, et al. Turn the World Upside Down—No One Notices

Actually, the first hint of what was going on came from Jeremy Morris's studies of London bus drivers. He was very concerned to make sure that his observations weren't messed up by what scientists call "confounding" variables, other things that you haven't looked at that might really be causing the phenomenon you are observing.

One of the questions he asked was whether body size made a difference. Fortunately, all the busmen wore uniforms that were issued to them by the London

Transit Authority and Morris got the Transit Authority, with the support of the busmen, to give him the trouser size of all the drivers and conductors.

And when he matched the trouser size up to their cardiac mortality rates, he discovered that weight didn't make any difference. The conductors still had half the cardiovascular mortality rates of the drivers, "whatever their physique—slim, average, or portly."[1]

But it took forever for the world to accept that fitlessness was a critical risk factor in all-cause mortality. And Morris's findings about weight were totally ignored.

The first epidemiological treadmill-based study that offered a glimpse of the huge impact that fitness had across all weight levels was Dr. Blair's 1989 research paper that we discussed in the previous chapter.[2]

The main purpose of that study was to conclusively prove that fitness reduced all-cause mortality. But it was a very thorough study that looked at a whole bunch of variables including smoking, cholesterol levels, blood pressure, family history, blood sugar levels, and weight.

And there was a big surprise. They discovered that heavy individuals who were fit had much lower death rates then unfit individuals who were thin.

This study was not really conclusive because the researchers were not focusing on the relationships among weight, fitness, and all-cause mortality, and because the BMI groupings they used were less than 20, 20 to 25, and over 25. But the findings sparked a flurry of research on the subject.

About BMI

Most studies classify weight using the BMI scale. You can find a BMI table in Appendix 1. BMI relates height to weight and produces a number. The table itself is non-judgmental. It is simply a constructed number.

To make a long story short (and we will go into this in more detail in Part V), the Weight Loss Industry hijacked a committee of the World Health Organization and got it to classify people who were BMI 25 to 30 as overweight. and people who were BMI 30 and above as obese. Shortly thereafter, the health bureaucracy in the U.S. bought into these classifications.

One study looked at a broader range of BMI values.[3] Another made sure that other potential confounding variables, such as previous illness, smoking, alcohol intake, etc., weren't fouling up the results.[4] One even looked at waist size and body composition to make sure that the problems with BMI itself (someone who is very muscular with very low fat levels can still have a very high BMI due to the way BMI is calculated) weren't affecting the results.[5]

And then a couple of researchers published a review of twenty-four different studies that had looked at the impact of weight and fitness, not only on all-cause mortality but also at death rates for a number of specific disease entities.[6]

In each case, the results revealed the same thing. Heavy people who were fit had substantially lower all-cause mortality rates (and death rates for a number of specific disease entities) than thin people who were unfit.

Then, in 1999, Dr. Wei and his team published the most comprehensive analysis on the topic to date in the *Journal of the American Medical Association.*[7] He and his team took a database of 25,714 men who had had a complete physical examination and a treadmill fitness test and followed them for a period of twenty-four years. All told, they had 258,780 person years of follow-up (by any standards, this was a huge study).

The following graphics show what they found. All-cause mortality rates for each BMI group are broken down by levels of fitness. For the BMI 25 and under group their findings paralleled what we already knew, namely that the all-cause mortality rate for people who are fit is reduced by more than 50 percent versus those who were not fit—1.0 versus 2.2. (Researchers generally pick one group, in this case the BMI under-25/fit group, as a reference point of 1.0. They then compare all the other groups to that group.)

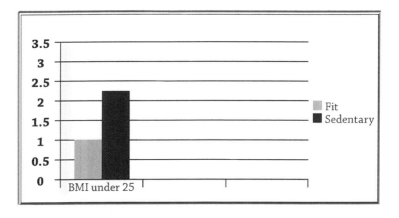

And when they looked at the higher weight levels for those who were not fit, the all-cause mortality rates increased relative to the lowest weight group that was fit (2.5 and 3.1 versus 1.0).

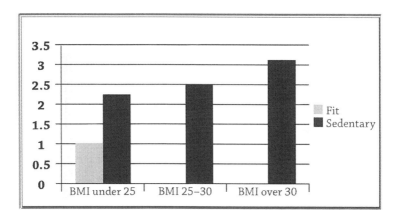

But then, when they looked at the heavier groups that were fit, they found that all the fit groups had essentially the same rates of all-cause mortality regardless of their weight (1.0, 1.1, and 1.1).

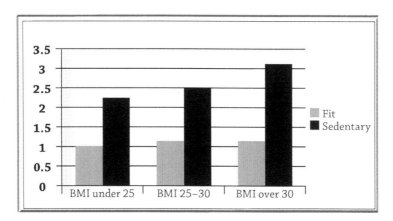

Bottom line: As long as you are fit, it does not matter what you weigh. But if you are not fit, being heavy compounds the problem. At BMI under 25, if you are not fit, you have at least twice the rate of all-cause mortality of anyone who is fit, regardless of his or her weight. If you are BMI 25–30 and not fit, you have 2.5 times the rate of all-cause mortality of anyone who is fit, and if you are BMI over 30 and not fit, you have about three times the rate of all-cause mortality of anyone who is fit.

If you are fit, it does not matter what you weigh. You will have the same lower rate of all-cause mortality regardless of your weight. And of course, when death rates drop, so do the rates of all the illness that can cause mortality. When you are fit, overall you are much healthier, regardless of your weight.

So, if you have a BMI of 25–30 and you are fit or a BMI over 30 and you are fit, what do you need to do to be healthy? **NOTHING!** You are in great shape. Just keep up your fitness routine.

But if you have a BMI of 25–30 or over 30 and are unfit, now what do you need to do to be healthy? Well, you have been told ad infinitum that you should lose weight. But will that do it for you?

Well, if you get your weight down to a BMI of 25, but you stay unfit, what have you got? Now you have only double the chance of dying that a fit person who weighs what you used to weigh has. Fantabuloso!

But what happens if you get fit, and stay the same weight? You reduce your chances of dying of anything by 60 percent if you have a BMI of 25–30 and by 68 percent if you have a BMI over 30. And getting fit enough to accomplish that is way easier than losing weight and keeping it off.

5

But How Can That Be?

This is all pretty mind blowing. People talk all the time about how bad fat is. Are you really saying that body fat is okay?

We've been conditioned to the mantra that body fat is bad, bad, bad. Guess what? Your body doesn't agree. Your body is adamant and tenacious in not agreeing. As far as your body is concerned, fat is good, good, good.

Why? Because in the couple of hundred thousand years that human beings have existed and in the millions of years of evolution leading up to human beings, feast or famine was a way of life. Your next meal was never certain and famine was always a very real possibility. So evolution invented an incredibly efficient means to store energy—fat. Without fat, we would not be here today. We would have died out long ago. Fat allows us to consume and store as much energy (food) as we can when it's available, so that we have energy to live off when it's not available.

A pound of fat is about 3,500 calories. It requires just about 100 calories to walk a mile. So let's say there is no longer any food here, but we know that there is food thirty-five miles from here. To walk from here to that food source, we only need to burn the energy in one pound of fat. Ten pounds of fat gives you enough energy to walk 350 miles.

But if your body loves fat so much, why does your all-cause mortality go up if you are heavy and unfit? The answer is that your body never expected you to be sedentary. Our body is tuned to move a lot. All of our evolutionary ancestors, and modern day humans up until several thousand years ago, were hunter-gatherers. That's how we found food for energy. If one is hunting and gathering, one is on the move a lot.[1]

Think of it this way. Every species has been fine-tuned by evolution to function best in a specific manner. Dogs need to move a lot. If they don't, it's not healthy for them. So you take your dog for walks. Try taking your cat for a walk. Even if you could somehow manage to get it to go for a walk with you, it probably wouldn't be good for it. That's simply not how cats are tuned.

Have you ever seen a sloth? I had the good fortune to see some in the wild in Panama. The word itself has taken on pejorative overtones, but in fact, sloths are really cool animals. They are probably the slowest moving animals on earth, but when they do move, they move in such an absolutely graceful dance, it is beautiful to watch. The sloths are fine-tuned to be stationary most of the time (they can sleep up to nineteen hours a day) and to move very slowly when they do move. For a sloth, that's healthy. That's sloth fitness.

Every species has its own definition of fitness. The human body is fine-tuned to move a lot and to burn a lot of energy every day. If we do that, we're fit. If we don't, we're not. Your body really, really wants you to be fit. Your body expects you to be fit. If you are fit and carrying around some extra stored energy, your body is very happy. And as we have seen, the death rate of people who are fit is almost identical regardless of their weight. But when you are not fit, you are really gumming up the works. The body doesn't know how to deal with Fitlessness. Fitlessness, even if you are thin, doubles your death rate. And the problem gets compounded when you are not fit and add additional weight to the equation.

So if you are carrying extra weight, you are not trapped! By getting fit, you can eliminate all of the negative health consequences that have been attributed to being heavy.

Okay, but everything I've ever seen or heard or read has said that in order for us humans to get fit, you have to exercise, you have to get your heart rate up, you have to sweat. But you keep saying that you can get fit enough without exercise. So how do you do that?

Piece of cake. It's all about movement and learning to walk—10,000 steps at a time.

6

If the Answer Is 10,000, the Question Is...?

But you can't get fit enough just by walking, can you?

Well, actually you can, because once again the received wisdom, what everybody knows, "just ain't so." And what is it that everybody knows? Well, the "aerobics revolution" led us to believe that the **ONLY WAY** to get fit is to get your heart rate up, to have a vigorous workout, to work up a sweat and to do it all at once without stopping.

The aerobics revolution really got underway with the publication of Dr. Kenneth Cooper's *Aerobics* in 1962[1] and the *Aerobics Way* in 1977.[2] He developed a point system and recommended that everybody accumulate thirty to fifty points of high intensity activity a week. And he provided charts, giving the points for all kinds of activities including running, cycling, handball, speed walking, swimming, skipping rope, stair climbing, etc.

And thus was born the aerobics doctrine. In 1975, the American College of Sports Medicine issued its first workout guidelines calling for all healthy adults to work out at aerobic intensity continuously for twenty to thirty minutes at least three times a week. The American Heart Association and the federal government adopted these standards more or less intact.

The problem with this was that although some people took up aerobic exercise and got very fit indeed, most people did not. To quote from an article in the *Harvard Men's Health Watch*, "The aerobics doctrine inspired the few but discouraged the many."[3] That level of highly intense vigorous activity was more than most people felt they could do, and as a result, they did nothing.

Fortunately, a number of researchers began to question whether vigorous aerobic workouts were the only way to obtain the benefits of being fit. And what they found was that workout intensity was NOT the determining factor. The determining factor was ***total energy expended.***

Now the good old law of conservation of energy tells us that if I have a block of metal weighing 140 pounds, and I want to move that block of metal one mile, I will more or less use the same amount of energy regardless of how fast I move it. If I move it a mile in ten minutes, I will use roughly the same energy that I would use if I moved it a mile in twenty minutes. If I move it faster, I will use more energy per minute, but the total energy used in moving it a mile will be roughly the same, regardless of speed.

Therefore, if you weigh 140 pounds (or 175 or 250) and you run a mile in ten minutes, you'll use roughly the same amount of energy that you would have used if you had walked that mile in twenty minutes. When you run, you burn more energy per minute than you do when you walk, but when you have covered that mile you will have burned about the same amount of energy regardless of whether you walk or run.

And so the idea that walking is a second-best, pale imitation of running or other aerobic exercise such as biking, swimming, in-line skating, aerobic dance, etc., is simply false, and there is extensive research that confirms this.

A study was published in the *New England Journal of Medicine* in 1999 by JoAnn Manson, et al., with the somewhat lengthy title of "A prospective study of walking as compared with vigorous exercise in the prevention of coronary heart disease in women." This study analyzed a database of over 72,000 women who had been followed for a period of eight years. The study concluded that "The magnitudes of risk reduction associated with brisk walking [20 minutes per mile pace] and vigorous exercise are similar when total energy expenditures are similar."[4]

In 2002, Dr. Manson analyzed a different database of over 73,000 women and came up with the same results.[5] Walking works!

If you think about it, the research makes intuitive sense. Our bodies are in fact fine-tuned for walking. As I mentioned in the last chapter, anthropologists estimate that primitive man walked many miles a day. Sure, our ancestors had brief bouts of high-energy expenditures, such as running away from tigers, hunting dinner, fighting with neighboring tribes, having sex, etc. However, for the most part, primitive man walked.

And this is true not only of humans but of most other animals as well, even those that are good runners such as horses or deer. They run occasionally, but mostly they walk.

Our bodies are fine-tuned for walking and that is how we function best. None of this is to say that jogging or swimming or biking aren't good too. They are all perfectly fine. It's just that walking is an equally effective way to get fit and stay fit.

Okay, so in order to get fit, how much do I have to walk?

Ideally, you'd like to walk an average of 10,000 steps a day.

Why use steps rather than minutes of walking? The recommendations I have seen are all over the lot. Some say you should do an hour a day. Others say half an hour most days of the week. But they all seem to concentrate on the amount of time you spend. Why do you focus on steps instead?

Okay, let's take a step back. The key to fitness is total daily energy expenditure. And although it may not seem like it, the overwhelming majority of our energy expenditure each day involves moving the weight of our bodies from here to there.

For example, let's assume that you have a large basement and that you have some shelves that line the walls. One of the shelves is about waist high, and on that shelf, going all the way around the basement, you have stored sixty-five boxes, each of which weighs fifteen pounds. You have decided to rearrange everything on the basement shelves, and one of the things you need to do is place those sixty-five boxes on the next shelf up. Each of the shelves is about a foot apart.

So you go down to the basement and spend about ten minutes lifting those boxes up on to the next higher shelf. Then you go up to the kitchen to get a glass of water.

Let's look at the total energy expended in this whole process. When you finished lifting those sixty-five boxes to the next shelf, you will have lifted a total of 975 pounds a distance of one foot. That was probably pretty tiring, unless you're used to doing that kind of work. Your arms might even feel a little sore.

Then you went upstairs. In most houses, floors are separated by approximately nine feet. If you weigh 155 pounds, when you walked upstairs, you lifted your entire body weight nine feet. This would be the same as if you had lifted nine boxes weighing 155 pounds each one foot from that lower shelf to the higher one. So when you walked up the stairs from the basement, you lifted a total of 1,395 pounds one foot. You did that in about seven to ten seconds and you hardly even noticed it.

Our legs are incredibly strong. They move our entire body weight constantly throughout the day. The overwhelming majority of the calories that we expend during the day involve moving our body from here to there. However, because our legs are so strong and because we are so used to moving about, we hardly even notice it.

Therefore, every step counts because every step expends energy. When you wear a pedometer (more on that in a minute) you get to count every step you take. And every step you take, regardless of what you are doing, counts toward making you fit.

The problem with using minutes rather than steps is that everybody's situation is different. If you are a nurse working on a busy hospital floor, there's a good chance that you'll be taking 700 to 800 steps an hour.[6] If you wait tables at a restaurant or deliver the mail on foot in an urban area, you also take lots of steps every day. And if you spend five hours at the mall doing Christmas shopping, you have taken a ton of steps. And all those steps count because each one of them involves energy expenditure.

On the other hand, if you are computer programmer or a customer service representative sitting at a desk all day, you're not going to get much in the way of steps at work.

As a result, the standard recommendations expressed in minutes are going to be more than necessary for the nurse, restaurant server, or mail deliverer and too little for the computer programmer or the customer service representative.

That's why counting steps is far better. You know exactly where you are every day and what you need to accomplish to meet your goals.

Okay, but how do you know that 10,000 steps is the right number? That seems awfully convenient. A nice round number with lots of zeros.

Pure coincidence. It just happens that the amount of energy we need to expend to be fit works out to about 10,000 steps. It works out regardless of whether you use an input model, i.e. what you do to get fit; or an output model, i.e. the results you achieve from that effort.

In 1986, Dr. Ralph Paffenbarger published a study in the *New England Journal of Medicine* that looked at the leisure-time physical activity levels of 16,936 Harvard alumni, aged thirty-five to seventy-four. In other words, he looked at what activities people did, such as running, playing sports, biking and other forms of exercise. The biggest reduction in all-cause mortality was for people who expended 2,000 calories a week in these activities. Above 2,000 calories, the benefits tended to level off.[7]

Ever since then, the expenditure of approximately 2,000 calories a week in leisure-time activities (the input) has been considered the gold standard. Most analyses assume that the average sedentary person still takes approximately 4,000 steps just as a natural part of daily living and the energy expenditure for those 4,000 steps is not counted in the 2,000 calories per week requirement. To achieve that additional 2,000 calories a week, one needs to expend approximately 300 extra calories a day. And 6,000 steps equals approximately 300 calories. So the 4,000 steps per day that are deemed just part of daily living, plus the extra 6,000 needed to expend an additional 300 calories per day, ends up giving you a total of 10,000 steps.

If you look at it from the output side (what level of fitness results from an input of 10,000 steps per day), walking 10,000 steps a day pretty much guarantees that you will build your aerobic capacity up to 9 or 10 METs. This is the fitness level that you need to achieve in order to cut your all-cause mortality by at least 50 percent, and to eliminate any negative health consequences of carrying extra weight.

What's a MET?

A MET is a shorthand yardstick for measuring aerobic capacity. One MET is the amount of oxygen that you use while you're sitting and watching TV. Basically, it measures the size of your body's aerobic engine. The bigger your aerobic engine, the more oxygen you can use, and thus the higher your peak aerobic capacity. And the researchers basically have it down to the point now where they can tell how much oxygen somebody is able to use based on how long they're able to continue walking on a standardized treadmill test.

If on a treadmill test you can reach at least the peak aerobic capacity of 9–10 METs, then you know you've cut your chances of dying of anything by at least 50 percent, regardless of how much you weigh (see the box at the end of the endnotes for Chapter 3 for more on treadmill tests and METs). And the available research makes it clear that anybody who walks 10,000 steps will almost certainly test out with a peak aerobic capacity of at least 9–10 METs.[8]

Another reason that we are really comfortable with the 10,000 step recommendation is that there is growing acceptance in the scientific community that 10,000 steps equals the level of energy expenditure needed for adequate levels of fitness. In other words, a lot of highly respected people think that that is a good number.

For example, Dr. Kenneth Cooper, who launched the aerobics revolution with his books, subsequently founded the Cooper Institute for Aerobics Research in

Dallas. Now you might think that because he created the aerobics doctrine, his institute would be "doctrinaire" about it. Not at all. In fact the researchers at the Institute have been in the forefront of rethinking what is required to be fit. Andrea Dunn, who is the director of the Institute's Project Active, says "We encouraged participants to shoot for at least 8,000 to 10,000 steps a day."[9]

In a 2004 paper, Catrine Tudor-Locke, a leading expert in the area, classified people who take 7,500 to 9,999 steps per day as "somewhat active" and people who take 10,000 steps per day and over as "active."[10] In a follow-up paper in 2008, with a lot more data in hand, she stated that, "The zone delimited by 7,500 to 10,000 steps per day is amassing support as evidence continues to accrue that health benefits can be realized and that acceptable public health recommendations are achievable within this zone."[11]

David Bassett, also an expert in the field, says that people need to "make a concerted effort to get to 10,000."[12]

Finally, lots and lots of researchers are using 10,000 steps per day as a key touchstone criteria for their research papers.[13].

And there you have it. All it takes to reduce your all-cause mortality by at least 50 percent and eliminate the health problems associated with carrying extra weight is to walk 10,000 steps a day. So let's talk about how you get to 10,000 steps a day.

Okay, you've made a pretty good case that we need to be somewhere in the 10,000 steps per day zone. And yes, health is important, and we all would like to cut our risk of dying in half. And maybe that's enough for some people.

But I think there's something that you just don't get. There are a lot of people who would say to you "Mike, the health stuff is really nice, but that's not what it's all about for me. You see..."

7

It's All about How I Look, Stupid

Everybody in this world seems to be obsessed with thin. Heavy people are looked down upon. They experience discrimination. So health is important, but it's not only about health. Some of us just want to be thinner.

Got it. Now that we have conclusively proven that fat is not a disease and that there are no negative health consequences associated with being heavy provided you are fit, where does that leave us?

Exactly. It's all about how you look in the mirror. Because, once you eliminate the negative health consequences of heaviness by becoming fit, weight becomes exclusively an

aesthetic choice.

So the first question is, can you move away from the "I've got to lose weight to look okay and to feel good about myself" point of view? I'm not saying that you should or shouldn't. That is your choice. But a lot of people have made the transition to accepting the body that they have, so it might at least be worth exploring.

The umbrella term for this approach is "Health at Every Size." The focus is on size acceptance, learning how to develop and trust your own healthy instincts about food and eating, adopting healthy and active lifestyles, and embracing size diversity.

An excellent, very comprehensive book on the subject is Dr. Linda Bacon's *Health at Every Size: the Surprising Truth about Your Weight*.[1] There are also lots of resources online that provide information and support for the Health at Every Size approach.[2]

Now, before you jump down my throat and tell me that's all just Pollyanna-ish wishful thinking, be aware that there is some pretty good scientific research backing up the Health at Every Size concept.

One study involved seventy-eight women, aged thirty to forty-five with BMI's at or above 30.[3] The women were assigned randomly to participate in a "LEARN Program for Weight Control" (a well-respected diet program) taught by a registered dietician, or in a Health at Every Size (HAES) program that focused on "body acceptance, eating behavior, nutrition, activity, and social support." The program lasted twenty-four weeks and was followed by twenty-eight weeks of aftercare and then an additional year of follow-up.

Neither group achieved long-term weight loss. The diet group achieved short-term weight loss, but then put most of the weight back on. The HAES group did not achieve weight loss because no attempt was made to lose weight in that group.

At the end of the study, all of the participants were assessed on a variety of measures including lipid levels, blood pressure, activity levels, eating behaviors, psychological mood, etc. The clear result was that at the end of the two-year study, the HAES group had substantial improvements in health risk indicators versus the dieting group.

Perhaps even more significant, in the evaluation forms that participants filled out at the end of the program, 100 percent of the HAES group said the program helped them feel better about themselves versus only 47 percent of the diet group. Only 5 percent of the HAES group felt like they had failed the program as opposed to 53 percent of the diet group. Perhaps most importantly, 89 percent of the HAES group reported that they were implementing the tools they learned in the program, whereas only 11 percent of the diet group said that they were implementing what they had learned in the program.

Other studies have confirmed the beneficial effects of the HAES approach.[4,5] Clearly, the Health at Every Size approach has worked well for many people and is worth serious consideration.

> *Okay, I agree, that is really good advice for some of us. But for some of us it just doesn't cut it. So we're closet fatistas. See, I admitted it. Some of us just plain don't want to be as heavy as we are right now. But if we start walking and get fit, will we lose weight? Is that the answer to everything?*

PART
II

POUNDS

Losing Them

Making Sure They Don't Find You Again

8

I Still Want to Take It Off,
I Want to Take It All Off

Got it. And just to make things really nice and complicated, there are actually four questions involved here.

1. Will you lose weight if you get fit?
2. Will getting fit and dieting at the same time result in your losing weight faster than if you just dieted alone?
3. Will fitness keep the pounds off if you do lose some weight?
4. Will fitness maintain your existing weight if you choose not to diet?

Let's look at the first question here and the others in the next few chapters.

We all know somebody, or know somebody who knows somebody, who went out, started a fitness program, lost a lot of weight without dieting and has kept it off ever since. We are so happy for them and we hate them.

In order to lose weight, you need to consume less energy than you expend. When you walk 2,000 steps, you burn approximately 100 calories of energy. A pound of fat stores 3,500 calories of energy.

Now let's say that before you started your fitness efforts, you averaged about 4,000 steps per day (which is pretty standard). You decide that you're going to increase that to 10,000 steps a day. So slowly and carefully (we'll talk a lot more about how to get there without overdoing it in a little bit) you work your way up to 10,000 steps. Now you are walking an extra 6,000 steps a day, so you are burning an extra 300 calories. After twelve days, you will have burned an extra 3,600 calories, or about a pound of fat.

If you do that, your weight should decrease by that amount, right? And if you kept doing that for a year, you would burn an extra 109,500 calories and so potentially, you could lose thirty-one pounds.

Will that happen? Well, that depends. Those few lucky folks who lost a lot of weight because of starting a fitness program managed to keep themselves from consuming an extra 300 calories of energy every day to make up that deficit. But these folks are very much the exception.

Carolyn Richardson et al. did a comprehensive review of studies that looked at what happened when people walked 9,000 to 10,000 steps a day but did not diet.[1] They looked at nine studies that met their strict inclusion criteria. In one eight-week study, participants actually gained about half a pound. However, in all the rest of the studies the participants lost weight. But the weight losses were very small.

In the shorter studies that lasted one to three months, the weight losses averaged about a pound a month. However, that level of loss tapered off as time went on and in the longer studies lasting six to twelve months, weight loss ranged between a half and three quarters of a pound per month.

So the answer is yes, you might lose a tiny bit of weight at first just by walking 10,000 steps. But you are extremely unlikely to lose a lot of weight, and any weight loss you do get will be in the first few months. After that, you will most likely level out.

So why is that? Here we are, burning 300 extra calories a day and yet we're likely to lose only minuscule amounts of weight, or not any at all. Why? It has to do with your body's set point mechanism. This mechanism is extremely fine-tuned. It tries to keep your energy input and your energy output in balance so that your weight stays even.[2]

Well, guess what? That regulatory mechanism, your set point, doesn't go on vacation when you start to get fit. When you start to burn more energy, your body notices. And what does your body tell you to do? It tells you to compensate for the extra energy you're burning so that you can keep your weight even. How does it tell you? It makes you hungry. So over the course of the day you eat an extra 300 calories to compensate, your body is happy, and your set point is working. And so, even though you might lose a little when you start your fitness program, over time, you'll almost assuredly stay at the same weight if you don't consciously try to diet.

9

Dieting and Fitness—Perfect Together?

The answer to the second question, will dieting and walking 10,000 steps result in your losing weight faster than if you just dieted alone is, it depends.

For example, in one study, participants agreed to maintain a super starvation diet of 1,000 calories per day over an eight-week period.[1] The participants were divided into a diet-only group and a diet and fitness group. As you can imagine, both groups lost a ton of weight. The diet-only group lost about twenty-two pounds or a whopping 2.75 pounds per week (ouch, too much per week). The diet and fitness group lost 26.5 pounds; a massive 3.3 pounds a week (double ouch, way too much per week).

Why did the fitness group lose more? Well, if both groups were only eating 1,000 calories per day and the fitness group was expending more energy than the diet-only group, of course the fitness group would lose more since they had a bigger calorie deficit. So when performed in a clinically controlled environment, the answer is yes, dieting and fitness causes one to lose more weight than just dieting alone.

But, would you want to do that? That depends on how you usually diet and what makes dieting difficult for you. If hunger is your biggest problem when dieting, it might make things more difficult.

Assuming that you have dieted in the past, you probably have a specific calorie deficit that you are comfortable using. For instance, if you normally achieve a weight loss of a pound a week, you have been working with a 500 calorie per day deficit (500 calories times seven days equals 3,500 calories or about a pound of fat).

Now let's say that you gradually increase your steps per day from 4,000 to 10,000. As a result, you will be burning an extra 300 calories each day. If you then go on a diet and you eat exactly the same amount that you always have on a diet, you will increase the calorie deficit to 800 calories per day (the 500 you are used to plus the 300 extra calories per day that you burn by walking the additional 6,000 steps per day).

Obviously, this will speed up your weight loss. But do you want to do that? If you suddenly jump up to an 800 calorie deficit by adding 300 calories of energy expenditure without compensating, all that's going to happen is that you will be even hungrier and it will make it that much harder for you to maintain your calorie limit.

So if hunger is your biggest problem when dieting, your best bet might be to stick with the calorie deficit that you're used to and add enough food calories to your diet to compensate for the 300 calories of extra energy you are expending by walking the extra 6,000 steps a day.

If, on the other hand, cravings and or feelings of deprivation are the biggest problems for you, and you don't get hungry or being hungry doesn't bother you, then the equation might change. You might decide not to compensate. Your feelings of deprivation would be no worse than usual, but with an 800 calorie deficit instead of a 500 calorie deficit, you get more weight loss for the same amount of deprivation pain.

Alternatively, you could go ahead and eat an additional 300 calories a day of yummy things and you would still lose weight at the same rate that you normally have in the past, but with fewer feelings of deprivation.

Another option is to do a stealth diet. If you are really good at maintaining your breakeven point and you don't get hunger pangs from dieting, then all you have to do is exactly maintain the calorie intake that was your breakeven point before you started walking the extra 6,000 steps a day. As you build up to 10,000 steps, your daily calorie deficit will increase, but you'll still be eating the same amount of food. In other words, you consciously avoid compensating for the 3,000 calorie deficit. No deprivation, no more cravings than usual.

Now you might say that the stealth approach is too slow because you're only losing at the rate of 300 calories a day, once you get up to 10,000 steps. But the trick here is that it won't feel like you're dieting. You'll be eating the same amount you always have. And 300 calories a day equals a pound in twelve days. If you religiously keep that up for a full year, you'll lose thirty-one pounds.

10

Are You the Energizer Dieter?

Before we go any further, I would like to ask you to take a little quiz. This quiz is only for dieters. If you have never dieted in your life, then you can skip this chapter and go on to the next one.

1. To the best of your ability to remember, how old were you when you went on your first diet?

   _____

2. What is your best guess as to what you weighed just before you started that first diet?

   _____

3. What is your best guess as to how many diets you've been on, or how much you have dieted since that first diet? If you only dieted three times in your life, then this is an easy question. If you diet a lot, you need to figure out some way to make a guess here. If you regularly go on three diets a year and it's been twenty years since that first diet, you would put down sixty diets. Alternatively, if you diet 50 percent of every year and it's been twenty years, then you might put down 520 weeks. Whatever works best for you.

   _____

4. What is your best guess as to the total number of pounds that you have lost since that first diet? Totally ignore pounds that you have gained back. In other words, if on three diets you've lost ten pounds each time, you would put down thirty pounds regardless of the fact that you might have gained them back. If you dieted two times a year for ten years and you lost fifteen pounds each time, put down 300 pounds.

   _____

5. What do you weight now?

   _____

Based on the answers to this quiz, let me ask you a question. Is losing weight really a problem for you? I suspect that for many of you the answer is no. In fact, for some people the answer to question four, the total number of pounds that you have lost is greater than the answer to question number five, what you weigh now.

So for many dieters the issue is not, "Can I lose weight?" The issue is...

11

I Don't Eat That Much—Why Can't I Keep the %#&*^# Weight Off?

Why can't you keep weight off after you've lost it? Very simple. Your body doesn't want you to. Your body has a set point. It's an equilibrium that it likes to maintain, that it considers to be good for you. It provides enough protection for you to ride out the occasional famine. The quarterback for managing the entire set point process is the part of your brain called the hypothalamus. It manages a whole complex battery of hormones and enzymes and other stuff in your body to keep you very close to that set point.

Now in the case of a real famine, your hypothalamus can't do much about it if there really is no food around. It will concentrate your mind on finding food by making you hungry. It will also get you to crave high-energy foods, and of course, the highest energy foods are the ones that are full of sugar and fat. But again, despite all its bag of tricks, if it is a real famine, the hypothalamus can't magically make food appear when it's not there. However, once the famine is over, the hypothalamus gets busy edging you back up to that set point.

When you diet, you are creating an artificial famine. Of course, your body can't tell the difference. As far as it's concerned, a famine is a famine. When you go off your diet, you try to avoid eating very much in order to maintain your weight loss. Your body sees that as a period of enough food, but not a lot of extra.

But your body is really smart and it's also tough as nails. When it can, it will sneak on a little extra here and a little extra there and slowly but surely, it will nudge your fat levels back up to that set point. It's on the job 24/7 and ultimately it gets you back to where it wants you to be, at your previous weight before the famine (diet). Why does it do that? Well, just in case there is another famine, you had better have those fat stores available if you want to survive. And your body is very tenacious about wanting you to survive the next famine.

You may have also noticed that after several attempts at dieting (experiencing multiple famines) and losing weight and putting it back on again, that you end up at a higher weight than when you started the diet process. In the quiz in the last chapter I asked you to put down your weight when you first dieted and your current weight. Is your current weight higher than the weight you were when you started dieting? For many people the answer is yes.

Why does this happen? The answer really is quite simple. Your body notices that you are experiencing a whole lot of famines (diets). Your body is really very strongly opposed to your starving to death. It gets the message that you live in a place where there are lots of famines.

Your body thought that it had some decent reserves to get you through a famine or two. But this is getting to be too much. What to do? Actually, it's really simple. Let's build some extra reserves so that if we suddenly have a bunch of famines in a row, we can ride them out. And so the body moves your set point up to a higher weight so that you have a larger fat reserve to make sure you survive all those famines (diets).

That is frighteningly discouraging. So what you're saying is that we are permanently trapped and that no matter how much we want to lose weight, there is absolutely no hope. But you know, there are some people who have lost weight and kept it off. And I'm not just talking about the nonsense you see on infomercials. I'm talking about real live people who I know or who are friends of friends who have managed to stay thinner. How did they do it if their body is so determined to move the set point higher after a diet?

Here's a little exercise. Write down in the left hand column of the box below the names of all those people. Then write down next to their name were kind of fitness activities they do.

If you don't know off the top of your head, give them a ring or ask them the next time you see them. Or if he or she is a friend of a friend, ask your friend what their weight-maintaining friend does for fitness.

Name	Fitness Activity

What you'll find, in almost every case, is that they are engaged in a continuous, ongoing fitness program. In fact, a major study by *Consumer Reports* in its June 2002 issue[1] surveyed over 32,000 dieters. Of those, 8,000 managed to lose 10 percent of their body weight and keep it off for one year. Of that group, 81 percent said that working out and being fit was a critical component of their being able to maintain their weight loss. These results track closely with those of the National Weight Control Registry, where 91 percent reported that staying fit was a critical component of maintaining weight loss.

Okay, so maybe I'm part of that small percentage of people who can keep weight off without fitness.

Sorry, but you are not part of that group.

What do you mean? How could you possibly know that?

Because we are having this conversation. If you had lost the weight that you wanted to lose and been able to keep it off without fitness, you would already have done so and we wouldn't be having this discussion. Therefore, I am 100 percent sure that if you lose some weight and you really want to keep it off, we simply have to start talking about keeping it off, 10,000 steps at a time.

12

Keeping It Off

Now this is really getting pretty monotonous isn't it? First it turns out that walking 10,000 steps cuts your risk of dying of anything by at least 50 percent. Then it turns out that walking 10,000 steps eliminates the health consequences of being heavy. And now it turns out that walking 10,000 steps is what you need to do in order to keep the weight off.

Honestly, this is for real. I didn't make this stuff up. I wouldn't dare. The science is absolutely unequivocal.

Now obviously, nothing works for everybody. And just as we might know somebody who lost weight by getting fit and didn't diet, we might also know some-body who is fit and still has trouble keeping weight off after a diet. However, the science and research is pretty conclusive that for the overwhelming majority of people, being fit and staying fit will result in their maintaining their weight loss after a diet.

The study I mentioned briefly in Chapter 9 gives some pretty dramatic proof of this. That was a study where the participants were put on a deep starvation diet of 1,000 calories a day and lost about three pounds a week. (Do not under any circumstances try this one at home.)

The participants in the study were divided into two groups. One group of dieters was told just to continue living as they had and asked not to participate in any physical activities or any fitness programs. The other group of dieters participated in a supervised fitness program. At the end of the program's eight-week diet phase, both groups had lost over twenty pounds (the fitness group a little more because both groups were eating the same number of calories, but the fitness group was expending more calories).

At the end of the diet phase, there was an eighteen month follow-up period. During the eighteen month follow-up, both groups were asked just to try to maintain their weight and not engage in any more dieting. The diet-only group was asked not to do any physical activity and the diet and fitness group was asked to continue its fitness regimen.

Based on a lot of research from many differ-ent studies, here is what we would expect to have happened. For the non-fitness group, we would ex-pect what could be called a lazy "V" shape that would look something like this:

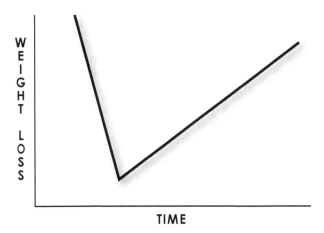

And that is, in fact, exactly what happened. The pattern for the non-fitness group exactly matches the lazy "V" pattern that we would expect. As soon as they went off their diets, the non-fitness group, slowly but inexorably, began to put the weight back on, even though they were trying to maintain their weight loss as best they could. And every dieter who has gone through the excruciating experience of con-stant weight cycling (also known as yo-yo dieting) can immediately identify.

Meanwhile, what is happening to the diet plus fit-ness group? What we would expect is that they would have what we might call an "L" pattern. Or perhaps, a little more accurately, a reclining "L" pattern that would look like this:

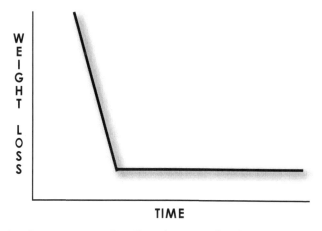

TIME

And sure enough, that is exactly the results that the investigators got. Once the fitness group ended their diet, they simply stayed where they were. Pretty conclusive, huh? The fitness group maintained their weight loss and the diet-only group went shooting back almost up to their previous weight.

But as they say in the infomercials, "Wait, there's more."

Sometimes, when people do research studies, some of the most interesting findings show up when the study participants don't do as they are asked. And that is exactly what happened with this study. A few participants in the diet-only group decided they would start a fitness program when the dieting phase of the experiment ended, never mind what the researchers asked them to do. And here is what happened to them.

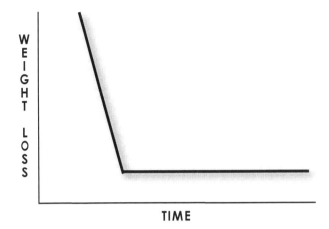

Yup. The exact same reclining "L" pattern that the original fitness group had. In fact, this small group of renegades actually lost a little more weight and then kept it off for the full eighteen-month period.

But wait, there's even more. Some of the folks in the fitness group decided to quit their fitness program at the end of the diet phase of the program. Well, what we would expect to see for that subgroup is that lazy "V" shape again.

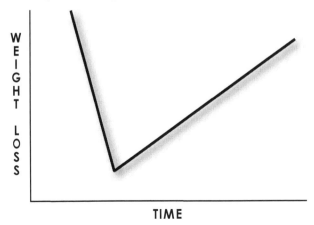

And yes, that is exactly what happened. The folks who quit the fitness program saw their weight gradually go back up, pretty much mirroring exactly what happened to the folks who were in the diet-only group.

And then there were even a few folks in the fitness group who kept their fitness regimen up for a few months and then quit. What would we expect the shape to look like for them? Probably something like a lazy "U." In other words, they kept the weight off as long as they stayed in the fitness program and then as soon as they quit, their weight began to move inexorably upward.

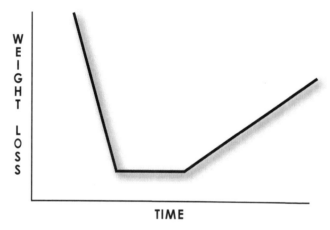

And yes, that is exactly what happened.[1]

And it is not just one study that has found this to be true. Many other studies have reached the same conclusion.[2-4]

Okay, so what is going on here? Based on what we said before about the set point, this shouldn't be happening. The body should be pushing everyone, including those in the fitness program, to regain weight. And it is successfully doing so with the diet-only, sedentary group. But that's not happening with the fitness group. Why not?

It turns out that the body actually has two set points accessible to it. Each set point is activated under a different set of circumstances. Now think of our ancestors for a moment. As we mentioned earlier, anthropologists believe that our ancestors walked a lot. That's a lot of energy expenditure. What were our ancestors doing, using up all that energy? Well, the answer pretty much has to be that, for the most part, they were looking for food, either hunting or gathering.

Now as far as your body is concerned, there's only one thing that's more important than having enough fat reserves to survive the next famine, and that's making sure that you don't have a famine in the first place. One of the problems with storing up extra fat to protect against future famines is that the more fat there is, the heavier you are, the more energy it takes to move your body to hunt and gather.

So your Internal Director of Storing Fat to Survive the Next Famine is somewhat in conflict with your Internal Director of Gathering Food to Make Sure That There Is No Famine in the first place. And they seem to have worked out a decent compromise.

When there is so much food around that you just don't have to move around very much to find it, then your Internal Director of Storing Fat gets to run hog wild and build up your fat reserves to guard against future famines. But when you start moving around a lot, it means that there is not that much food easily at hand and you have to move around to find it— hunting and gathering. In those circumstances, your Internal Director of Gathering Food has more clout. Not enough clout to convince the Fat Storing Director to give up much, if any, of the fat energy reserves that you already have built up, but enough clout to keep you from putting on any more weight that would require you to burn more energy as you look for food.

And so, as a result, there is an alternate set point, a fitness set point, that is activated because what we call fitness, your body interprets as critically needed activity to find food. Therefore, your body is willing to not encumber you with more weight so that you spend extra energy looking for that food.

Thus, if you diet but you don't get fit, you are condemned to an eternity of Sisyphean frustration. You'll go through the tortures of losing weight and then that rock rolls right back down to the bottom of the hill and you have to start all over again.

Fitness changes the whole equation. Sisyphus can be banished once and for all. You lose the weight that you want and you keep it off. Or, if your weight loss goals are more than can be accomplished with one diet, then you simply stop when you reach a plateau or you just can't stand it anymore. Then you just stay there for a while until you're ready to roll that rock up the hill some more. But it's never going to roll back on you.

13

10,000 Does It Again

Now, let's look at the last question. Will fitness help you maintain your existing weight if you choose not to diet? Yup. Absolutely. No question about it.

If you can activate your fitness set point by walking 10,000 steps a day after you diet, it just stands to reason that you can activate your fitness set point by walking 10,000 steps a day, whether you just came out of a famine (diet) or not. Your body still assumes you're looking for food and your Internal Director of Gathering Food takes control of the situation and makes sure that your Internal Director of

Storing Fat doesn't sneak in there and dump some extra weight on you, forcing you to use more energy to gather that food.

This was all borne out by a comprehensive study published in 2010 in the *Journal of the American Medical Association*.[1] But boy oh boy, it is simply mind-boggling how the world's most brilliant researchers can sometimes be the world's dorkyist communicators.

The headlines screamed exercise, **Exercise**, **EXERCISE**. The *LA Times* shouted "Women Should Exercise an Hour a Day to Maintain Weight, Study Says"[2] *The Cleveland Leader* thundered "Study: Women Who Don't Diet Should Exercise 1 Hour Per Day, 7 Days a Week."[3] *Businessweek* proclaimed "Women Must Exercise an Hour Each Day to Stay Lean, Study Says."[4]

And what was the reaction? Totally, 100 percent predictable. The response was, "No way. I don't have time for that." And then there was the study's director, who did nothing but add fuel to the fire by saying "There's no sugar coating it." "It's a large amount of activity. If you're not willing to do a high amount of activity, you need to curtail your calories a lot." In other words, either diet for the rest of your life or exercise for an hour a day. There was only one tiny, itty bitty, little problem with all of this.

THAT IS NOT WHAT THE STUDY SAID

What the study actually said was that women who expended at least 21.5 MET hours a week in physical activity, above what they would expend if they were sedentary, did not gain any weight.

So what's a MET hour?

Well, we have talked about using METs as a way to measure peak aerobic capacity. But it is also a really nice standardized tool to measure energy use in physical activity. As you will recall, one MET is the amount of energy that you burn when you are sitting watching TV.

When you sit and watch TV for an hour, your energy expenditure is one MET hour. The study said that if you expend 21.5 MET hours a week over and above what you would expend in normal, sedentary day-to-day living, about 4,000 steps a day for most people, you won't gain any weight.

Ten thousand steps to the rescue. Again assuming that the average, sedentary person walks about 4,000 steps a day, someone needs to add 6,000 steps to get to 10,000 steps a day.

Guess what? When you walk 6,000 steps, either all at once or in bits and pieces throughout the day, you burn about 3 MET hours of energy. Multiply that by seven and now you have 21 MET hours of physical activity per week.

One would really think that by now the research community would've figured out that for the majority of the population, "exercise" is an eight-letter dirty word, and that everybody and their brother and sister will immediately shut down and stop listening once they hear it.

When I give speeches on fitness and weight issues, I ask everybody who exercises regularly (by however they define "exercise" and "regularly") to please stand up. Between 10 percent to 20 percent of the people in the room stand up.

Then I say "If you like exercise or in some way find it satisfying or fulfilling, please raise your hand." Everybody who is standing (the exercisers) raises their hand as do a few people who are sitting. Then I say "If you are not exercising now because of an injury or illness or because life happens and you just can't do it right now, but you plan to get back into it as soon as possible, please stand up." Invariably, the people who were seated but had their hands raised now stand up. And equally telling, nobody who hasn't raised their hand stands up.

The bottom line is that those who like exercise or find it satisfying and fulfilling in some way are exercising or plan to get back into it as soon as possible. Those who don't like exercising, which is usually between 80 percent to 90 percent of the people in the room, aren't exercising now and have absolutely no intention of doing so in the future.

This should not really be a great revelation. People do things they like to do and avoid things they don't like to do. If I like chocolate ice cream, that's what I'll eat. If I don't like chocolate ice cream, I'll choose another flavor.

So what an incredible lost opportunity. What if the title of that study had read "10,000 Steps a Day Prevents Weight Gain over the Long Term"? And what if, as a result, the headlines had proclaimed, "Walking 10,000 steps a day keeps the weight away"?

Oh well. The bottom line is still the bottom line. Walking 10,000 steps a day is enough physical activity to turn on your fitness set point, and empower your Internal Director of Gathering Food to keep your Internal Director of Storing Fat from sneaking more weight on to you as the years go by.

So I can just eat whatever I want, whenever I want, and if I walk 10,000 steps, I'll never put on another pound, right?

You know, there is one basic rule for living life successfully. That rule is "you're never allowed to not think." Obviously, if you binge every day, and don't pay attention, you're going to put on weight. That's true whether you're just maintaining weight or trying to avoid regaining weight after a diet. But if you pay attention and try to maintain your weight, 10,000 steps a day will make it possible.

Okay, fine. But there's one other thing that's bothering me. Yes, it does seem that 10,000 steps is in the right zone for maintaining health and avoiding weight gain. But when you look at some of the details, and yes, I've looked at some of your endnotes, there seems to be a spread as to what's needed. So what is exactly the right number of steps that we need to take each day?

Research can be infuriatingly frustrating that way. The problem is that the studies are never exactly identical. They use different populations; they have different ways of measuring physical activities; they use different groupings of people; and they have different statistical techniques. As a result, it is really tough to compare apples to apples. Sometimes you're comparing apples to oranges, and every now and then you're comparing apples to pianos.

Ten thousand steps is absolutely in the right zone. There's just too much data revolving around that level of activity for anybody to really seriously question that that is where you need to be. But if you want real precision, then you're going to have to do some research.

Oh, give me a break, what do I know about research?

Granted, research is complicated when you're dealing with large numbers of people. However, here you'll only need to do research on just one person: you. You see, your body is different from anyone else's body. And so really, all you care about is how your body reacts to 10,000 steps a day.

And that is relatively simple to figure out. For the issue of maintaining weight or avoiding weight regain, here's what you need to do. Build yourself up to 10,000 steps, maintain a healthy diet, don't binge (except of course for Sunday brunch, and then skip supper) and weigh yourself from time to time. The likelihood is that your weight will hold steady. If it creeps up a little bit, then *your* body may require a few more steps above 10,000 to properly activate your activity set point. No problem, just add some steps until everything falls into balance and your weight holds steady.

With regard to your peak aerobic capacity, 9 METs to 10 METs is pretty much the magic zone you want to shoot for in order to cut your chances of dying from anything by at least 50 percent and to eliminate any negative health consequences of carrying extra weight.

Testing for this is a little tougher. You will need to take a treadmill test. So again, build yourself up to 10,000 steps and then maintain that for several months. Once that's totally comfortable and normal for you, then you can take a treadmill test to see if that is in fact producing a maximum aerobic capacity of 9–10 METs for you.

A treadmill test is relatively simple. An example of a commonly used treadmill test is the Balke protocol. You can find a copy of the protocol in Appendix 2. The protocols are a bit different for men and women, but they are basically the same. Throughout the test the speed remains the same (3.3 mph for men and 3.0 mph for women) but the incline will be increased as time goes on so you'll be walking more and more uphill, but at the same speed.

The longer you can manage to keep going, the higher your maximum aerobic capacity. If you look at the chart in Appendix 2, you will see that if a man can continue for a full fourteen minutes, he will have achieved 10 METs. If a woman can continue for a full twenty-two minutes (the buildup is more gradual for the female protocol), she will have achieved 10 METs.

If you reach those levels, then you are fine. If you fall a bit short, make an estimate as to how many additional steps you will need to do in order to get to 9–10 METs and then just increase your steps gradually to that point. Then after a while, take another treadmill test.

For most people, I think it's safe to just say walk 10,000 steps and everything will work. But if you really, really, want to know exactly and precisely where you stand, then that's the individual research you are going to need to do.

PART
III

Getting from Here to 10,000

14

Getting to 10,000

It does not matter how slowly you
go as long as you do not stop.
Confucius

The first thing you need to do is to buy one small
piece of equipment, a pedometer. You hook it onto
your waist on either side, just in front of the hip bone,
and it will count all the steps you take in a day. You
can buy a perfectly good one for between $10 and $30.
(If you want to spend a lot more money, you can also
get ones that will do the laundry, mind the kids, and
walk the dog.)

Put it on in the morning and keep track of all the steps you take each day.

The first week is simply for establishing your baseline. Don't do anything differently. Just go about your normal routine. Keep track of your steps for each day and write them in the Base Week Log below. Each morning, note how you feel and mark that in the log for the prior day. At the end of the first week, take an average of the three days with the highest step count where you also indicated that you felt good the next morning.

Base Week	Number of Steps	How Did You Feel the Next Morning?				Notes
		Good	Tired	A Little Sore	Very Sore	
Sunday						
Monday						
Tuesday						
Wednesday						
Thursday						
Friday						
Saturday						

For example, your base week might look something like this.

Base Week	Number of Steps	How Did You Feel the Next Morning?				Notes
		Good	Tired	A Little Sore	Very Sore	
Sunday	6,586			✔		Worked outside, raked leaves
Monday	3,452	✔				Normal day at work
Tuesday	4,268	✔				Normal day at work
Wednesday	6,102			✔		Went for a walk at lunch
Thursday	3,012	✔				Normal day at work
Friday	4,894		✔			Three meetings offsite
Saturday	9,875				✔	Heavy duty shopping at mall

The three highest step count days where you didn't feel tired or sore the next morning were 3,452, 4,268 and 3,012. Average the three days and you get 3,577. Round that off to 3,500 and that is your baseline. Then add 500 steps to the total to get 4,000. Your goal now is to get up to 4,000 steps a day. Once you get to 4,000 steps, stay there until that level of walking feels really comfortable. Then add another 500 steps per day and just keep doing that until eventually you work your way up to 10,000 steps.

Now, to make this happen, there are five key rules you must follow.

1. Take it slowly
2. Take it slowly
3. Take it slowly
4. Be patient
5. Take it slowly

The key is to listen to your body. Some days you may feel tired. Take a day off. If you push a little too much and feel a little sore, take a day off. The older you are, the more slowly you may need to go at the start. So what? This is a lifelong project. It doesn't matter if it takes you ten weeks, or thirty weeks, or two years to get to 10,000 steps, just as long as you get there and stay there.

The best way to start out is to do little things to add steps every day. Try parking at the far end of the parking lot at work. Basically, you take about 100 steps a minute. If it takes you an additional two and a half minutes each way to get to and from your car, then you just automatically added 500 steps a day. Try parking farther away at the mall and at the supermarket. It's just a matter of thinking, okay, how can I add another hundred steps here and another hundred steps there, and before you know it you'll have that extra 500 steps.

That will work like a charm for a while. But once your step count starts to get up there, you're going to need to take what I call "intentional walks." These can be very short walks of just five minutes or they can be longer walks. It doesn't matter as long as you get the steps in.

At work, you can take a walk during lunch or a walk during a coffee break. I've seen people walking while they are on business calls using their cell phone. If you have a fitness center at work and you have to listen to a conference call, go down to the fitness center, turn your cell phone to mute, and walk on a treadmill while you listen to the conference call. Convince your boss of the benefits of walking and every now and then have a walking meeting rather than an office meeting.

At home, you can walk on the street (quiet back streets without too much traffic are best). If your local school has a track, that's a good place to go. The local mall is also a good place to go, especially because many of them open early in the morning specifically to accommodate walkers.

Your local park may have walking trails and there may even be longer rail trails or canal towpath trails that are nearby. Google maps recently teamed up with the Rails to Trails Conservancy to show the locations of biking and walking trails throughout the country.[1] The homepage for these maps starts in San Francisco as of this writing, but as with any Google map, you just zoom out and move over to the portion of the country where you live and zoom back in again.

You can also walk indoors at home with a treadmill. Many people watch television or even read a book while they're walking. Now you may think that a treadmill is very expensive, and if you want a fitness center-quality treadmill, that's true. They will cost in the $4,000-$5,000 range. But those treadmills are designed to take a lot of abuse. They are used seven days a week and frequently they are used by runners.

All you will need is a walking treadmill and you can buy a perfectly good one for under $1,000, which is probably less than the cost of the TV that you're watching while you use the treadmill. You can also usually find used treadmills on craigslist.com for between $100 and $200.

What can you do while walking outside?

1. Talk to a walking partner
2. Listen to music
3. Listen to the radio
4. Talk on a cell phone
5. Plan your vacation
6. Think
7. Endless other possibilities

What can you do while walking inside on a treadmill?

1. Watch TV
2. Read
3. Listen to music
4. Listen to the radio
5. Talk on a cell phone
6. Think

But remember. Take it slow. Only add 500 steps a day at a time. Don't add more steps until you are comfortable at your new level. If you try to rush it you will get sore and tired, it will make you grumpy, and you will quit.

It also doesn't matter how fast you go. You'll probably start out somewhat slowly, but as you get stronger and more used to walking, your pace will naturally speed up.

So go slow, be patient, have fun, and you will absolutely get there.

Okay. That's wonderful. I know I may sound like I'm a bit of a pest here, but you really are missing something important. It's not only about the physical part of walking. For some people, there's a real body image psychological barrier here. And those people are going to say to you...

15

You Don't Understand, It's Embarrassing

Okay, it's time for a little grammar 101. The words embarrass and humiliate can really ONLY be used in a passive mode. Some words can be used both actively and passively. You can say "I was kissed" (passive mode), but for you to be able to say that, someone has to give you a kiss (active mode).

You can give someone a kiss (active mode), but you can't give someone a humiliate or an embarrass. You may feel humiliated or embarrassed by something someone did or said, but only you can create, inside your head, that feeling of humiliation or embarrassment. No one can do it to you. Therefore, you have a choice and you have control.

Let's say you go for a walk. And let's say that you walk down the street that is not too busy but has some traffic and also a few pedestrians. Maybe during your walk you will pass or be passed by about 200 people, most in cars, a few on foot.

Of the 200 people who see you on your walk, the likelihood is that none of them know you. Maybe twenty of them will actually notice you. Of those, ten will probably have a positive thought like "That person is really working on getting fit. Good for him or her." And maybe ten will have a negative, derisive, or prejudiced thought.

Do you really care either way? You don't know them, they don't know you, so it makes no difference.

Now let's say instead that as you walk you see someone whom you do know. And let's say that for this person, you actually do care what they think about you and what you're doing. One way to deal with this is to go up to them and sound them out to find out what they're thinking.

You might say something like, "Hi, Phyllis. I'm taking a fitness walk. Are you one of those brilliant, open-minded people who think that it is wonderful that I am doing that and you are so proud of me? Or are you one of those fatista jerks who is laughing her head off because you can't imagine how somebody who is heavy could possibly ever be fit?"

Well okay. You probably wouldn't do that. In fact, you probably wouldn't say anything close to that. But on the other hand, don't be shy either. Simply assume that they are one of those brilliant, open-minded people (because if they aren't, they'll never admit it anyway), and proclaim and own what you are doing. Tell them what you are doing and why you are doing it. Explain to them that people who are fit have the same chance of dying regardless of their weight, and the people who are not fit, regardless of their weight, at least twice the chance of dying as anybody who is fit.

Or, if you really want to blow their mind, here's something you can memorize.

"As you probably know, Dr. Wei and his research team published a study in 1999 in the *Journal of the American Medical Association* titled "The Relationship Between Low Cardiorespiratory Fitness and Mortality in Normal-weight, Overweight, and Obese Men." That study showed conclusively that heavy people who are fit died at half the rate of people who are BMI 25 or less and not fit, and that's why I'm out here working on my 10,000 steps a day fitness regimen."

You might also wear a T-shirt that says, "Come join me on my fitness walk," or "I'm walking 10,000 steps, can you keep up with me?" or if you really are feeling your oats it might say, "I can walk faster and farther than you can."

But whatever you do, stand up and be proud of it.

And, if in spite of everything I just said, your reaction is that you still just can't bring yourself to do it outside, at least until you get your step count up a little bit, then think about getting a treadmill to use at home. As I mentioned a moment ago, a perfectly good walking treadmill can be had for under $1,000, and you can usually find used treadmills on craigslist .com for between $100 and $200.

> *Okay, but just one more thing. We all lead horrendously busy lives. And much as we would like to do all that, a lot of people are going to say to you...*

16

I Simply Don't Have the Time

Okay, let's talk about time. Time is the most democratic of resources. We all have the same amount and we all have all there is.

Now you might expect me to say that the way to deal with the time problem is to make getting fit a high priority.

But the trouble with making getting fit a really high priority is that sometimes, often, amazingly more often than you might think, something seems to come along that has an even higher priority and bumps fitness out of the way. So priorities are really not going work that well.

There is another answer though. The answer has a sort of obvious, "well duh" quality to it. But it is so powerful.

Here's how it works. Have you ever been in a situation where you had to drop a child off at school or pick the child up from school every day? Would you characterize dropping the child off or picking the child up as something that had a high priority? Probably not, because if it only had a high priority, other priorities could come along and bump it out of the way. "Gee Sally, I'm really sorry I wasn't able to pick you up today at school. Something at work came along that had a higher priority. I hope hitchhiking home in the rain was a formative experience for you."

Not likely!

So picking up your child wasn't a priority, it was a **REQUIREMENT**. It simply had to get done every day, day in and day out. It was something that other things were scheduled around.

There may not be enough time in the day to fit in all the priorities, but there is always enough time for those few things in your life that are requirements.

So if you want to get fit and stay fit, then walking 10,000 steps must become a REQUIREMENT in your life, something that other things are scheduled around, something that simply has to be done. As they would say on *Mission Impossible* "**your mission, should you choose to accept it, is to make getting fit and staying fit a requirement in your life.**"

And if you do that, then you do something fundamental. You make a real commitment to get fit and then you **WILL** get fit.

17

Dealing with a Visit to the Doctor

This is just a bit off topic, but it keeps coming up so let's deal with it. Some people resist going to see the doctor because they are sick of the "You need to lose weight" lecture they get.

Don't do that. If you need to see the doctor, go. And don't skip your annual checkup. Just develop a strategy for dealing with the issue.

First of all, stop being mad at your doctor. The weight-loss lecture is in fact a sign of caring, because your doctor believes that carrying extra weight is detrimental to your health. Which would you rather have? A doctor who cares and brings it up, or a doctor who doesn't care or who is too timid to discuss it with you?

The problem is simply that your doctor is not well educated on the matter. So, assuming that you've decided to accept your body weight as it is and get fit by walking 10,000 steps, here are some suggestions. (This discussion isn't relevant if you have decided to take weight off and then keep it off by walking 10,000 steps.)

Basically, what you need to do is to bring your physician up to date on the actions you're taking and educate him or her as to the scientific evidence that supports what you are doing. You should probably bring three or four things with you to your visit.

These would be your step log, Dr. Wei's article showing that fitness eliminates the negative health consequences of carrying extra weight (endnote 7 in Chapter 4), Dr. Kokkinos' article showing the impact of fitness on all-cause mortality (endnote 6 in Chapter 3), and perhaps Dr. Bacon's study on health at every size (endnote 4 in Chapter 7).

Then, take the initiative early on and bring the whole subject up yourself. Go over your step log and review your progress to date (if you are not at 10,000 steps yet) or demonstrate the fact that you have maintained 10,000 steps on a consistent basis for a while.

Then give your physician a copy of Dr. Wei's article (make sure to use a marker to highlight the key last two lines of data in Table 2 on page 1,550) and explain its relevance, and then do the same with the other two articles.

This will totally change the discussion. You are now a partner in managing your health and you are demonstrating a level of expertise in this area that your physician probably does not have.

If all else fails, suggest that your physician send you for a treadmill test (if you've already reached 10,000 steps or, if you are not there yet, do it when you have reached 10,000 steps) so that you can demonstrate the level of aerobic capacity that you have achieved.

PART
IV

Everything Else the Weight Loss
Industry Doesn't Want You to Know

18

Introduction

The Weight Loss Industry is neither moral nor im-
moral. It is simply amoral. It does what every industry does, which is seek to increase revenue and
profits in any way it can.

The biggest danger to Weight Loss Industry profits is fitness. The big players in the industry all have
planning and research departments. They know in
great detail about all of the research that we have
been discussing. And they know exactly how dangerous that research is to their bottom line.

They know that if a whole lot of people who are
heavy begin a 10,000 steps a day fitness program in

order to get healthy, and then decide that they are comfortable with their body size after all, they won't need the services of the Weight Loss Industry anymore. That's massive demand erosion.

They also know that a 10,000 steps a day fitness program will prevent weight regain for the overwhelming majority of people. A huge amount of the demand for the services of the Weight Loss Industry comes from repeat customers—people lose weight, gain it back, lose it, gain it back, and so on indefinitely. But if people lose weight, begin a 10,000 steps a day fitness program, and as a result don't gain the weight back, another huge chunk of demand falls by the wayside.

Even worse, if people who are not heavy now begin a 10,000 steps a day fitness program and keep at it for the rest of their lives, the overwhelming majority of them will never gain weight and therefore never even be potential customers for the Weight Loss Industry.

Therefore, fitness is the most serious potential threat facing the profitability of the Weight Loss Industry.

How the Weight Loss Industry has managed to bury the real truth about weight and fitness with an avalanche of Researchaganda and what we can do about it is something we will focus on in Part V.

However, first let's look at the various players that make up the Weight Loss Industry and some things they would very much prefer you not know.

19

Committing Hari Kari—Non-Fatal (Mostly) Version

Hari kari surgery works by reducing the size of your stomach, either with a gastric bypass, by placing a band around the top part of the stomach or by other similar means.[1] As a result, you have a much smaller stomach, so you can't eat as much at one time, so you eat less and you lose weight.

The official name for this surgery is Bariatric (Barry–@–Rick).

And you can prove to yourself that this type of surgery works. Just cut out a piece of your stomach and you will find that you experience an immediate loss of appetite.

Hari kari surgery is a very, very big business. Marketdata Enterprises[2] reports that in 2006 there were 177,000 hari kari surgeries performed, a record. The total cost of those surgeries was $4.4 billion or roughly an average of $25,000 per surgery.[3]

The laparoscopic banding part of the business (where a flexible band is used to create a small pouch at the top of the stomach that needs to be adjusted on a regular basis) is expanding rapidly as medical entrepreneurs open freestanding and hospital-based banding centers.

Hari kari surgery is touted as a medical procedure designed to reduce your risk of dying by conquering the "disease" of obesity. Well, in the first place, as we have seen, obesity is not a disease. Secondly, this procedure has real risks. Although surgical death rates have improved somewhat over the years, a patient's chance of dying within thirty days of the operation is approximately 1 to 2 percent. That's one or two deaths in every 100 operations. If a surgeon is inexperienced with the procedure, those deaths rates can go as high as 5 percent.[4]

And even if you do survive the procedure, complication rates are huge. One study found that the complication rate was 39.6 percent during the 180 days after discharge.[5] A longer-term study followed laparoscopic banding patients for a period of thirteen years. The study found that "nearly 50 percent of the patients required removal of their bands." The study concluded that the procedure "appears to result in relatively poor long-term outcomes."[6]

Even some people in the weight loss business have voiced concern about the overselling of hari kari surgery. "Because it's risky, it's only appropriate for a tiny fraction of people with obesity—the sickest 1 to 2 percent," says Dr. Kaplan (director of the Massachusetts General Hospital Weight Center in Boston), "The idea that all obese people should get surgery is insane."[7]

Anyone seriously considering bariatric surgery absolutely must do their own homework. The folks selling the surgery may not present the full range of risks and complications a patient is likely to encounter. Fortunately, a number of websites provide a more complete information set. One such is the Obesity Surgery Information Center.[8] A Google search will turn up many more.

If one survives the surgery and avoids major complications, some research seems to show that people who undergo the procedure do reduce their mortality rates. These studies suggest that there are reductions in all-cause mortality of between 33 percent and 34 percent versus those who have not had the surgery.[9,10] However, a more recent study, with much more rigorous statistical controls, found no improvements at all in all-cause mortality.[11]

But why undergo risky, life-altering surgery when fitness alone can produce far better results? Remember the study by Dr. Wei. Here is the graphic again showing the results of that study.

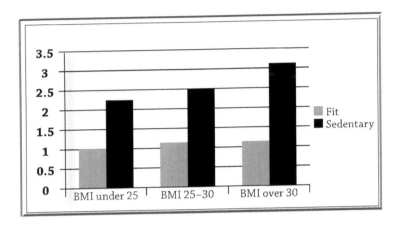

Now this study only went to BMI 30 and above. Although there is no good data splitting the BMI 35–40 and BMI over 40 population (who are the weight groups currently eligible for the surgery) between fit and sedentary, it's probably safe to assume that people who are BMI 35 and over and sedentary have an all-cause mortality that is somewhat higher than people who are BMI 30 and over and also sedentary. Let's make a guess that their all-cause mortality would be four times higher than the fit group.

Assuming all goes well and they survive the surgery, they might or might not reduce their all-cause mortality some (depending on which study you accept), but they will still have an all-cause mortality that is at least two and a half times that of the fit group.

But now, let's say that they chose not to have hari kari surgery but instead decided to start a 10,000 steps a day walking program. Their all-cause mortality would then drop not by 33 percent, but by about 75 percent.

Now of course, if the person who underwent surgery also decides to get fit, then they will have the same rate of all-cause mortality as everyone else on the chart who is fit. But then, why go through all the agonies of the surgery when you could have achieved the same health benefit by just walking 10,000 steps a day?

But can someone that heavy really get into a walking program successfully?

Why not? Someone who is 5'6" and weighs 247 pounds is at a BMI 40 level. Someone who is six-foot and weighs 294 pounds is also at BMI 40. Granted, that is heavy, but most people can walk without a problem at that weight.

The only time that hari kari surgery becomes a clear medical necessity is for that extremely small group of people who are so heavy that they can no longer walk, or for whom walking is so painful, because of the pressure on their knees and feet, that they would never be able to achieve 10,000 steps.

So if hari kari surgery is not a medically required procedure, what is it?

It is cosmetic surgery, and high-risk cosmetic surgery at that.

Let's be clear. That is **not** a pejorative, negative, value-laden statement. We are, each of us, in charge of our own bodies. We have the absolute right to do whatever it is we wish to do to change our appearance in any way that is pleasing to us. If doing so involves cosmetic surgical intervention, that is our decision and we are absolutely entitled to make that decision. But one should only do it with their eyes wide, wide open because the risks are serious and real.

Hari kari surgery is also often touted as an escape from dieting. A recent Google search for "Lap Band billboard images," turned up pictures of billboards that say things like "Dieting sucks." The implication is that if you have the surgery, you can be thin without dieting.

Nothing could be further from the truth. Hari kari surgery is not magic pixie dust. Hari kari surgery cuts your stomach down to a much, much smaller size. Your new, tiny stomach forces you to diet. And it forces you to diet, 24/7, forever. And many people find it difficult or impossible to adjust to the dramatically and permanently altered eating patterns that are required after the surgery.

Hari kari cosmetic surgery is a huge and profitable business and eligibility levels have now been shoved way down. People who are just BMI 40 and over, and people who are BMI of 35 and over with so-called "co-morbidities" are now eligible for hari kari cosmetic surgery (a co-morbidity means that you have some other disease entity.)

And that's not the end of it. In February of 2011, Allergan, a maker of gastric bands, succeeded in getting FDA approval to use its device on patients with a body mass index of 35 without co-morbidities, and on people with a BMI of 30 who have co-morbidities.

That would mean that a woman who is 5'6" and weighs 186 pounds or a man who is six-foot and weighs 221 pounds would be eligible for hari kari surgery.[12]

That's crazy. Isn't there something that we can do about that?

Unfortunately, we can't. I mean, what are we going to do, march on Washington? Waste of time. Yes, we can work collectively to change the public perception of weight issues, and we will talk a lot about that later on. But on specific cases like this, there is no real way to control the outcome. Hari kari surgery is a very big business. This new expansion down to BMI 30 could mean billions of dollars of additional profit for the hari kari industry.

Ultimately, the only way to stop this is through individual action.

How can we stop it individually?

Well, look at the case of the Decorative Scarring Centers of America.

The who?

The Decorative Scarring Centers of America. You know, in some cultures decorative scarring is a mark of great bravery and distinction. A decorative pattern is carved into the skin and then various herbs and other things are rubbed into the cut so that when it heals it will produce a raised, decorative scar. And of course, all this is accomplished without any type of anesthesia or sedation or even liquor. That's why it's considered a mark of bravery.

That's gross. Anyway, there are no Decorative Scarring Centers of America.

That's right, and why do you think that is?

Because no one in their right mind would do that.

Exactly. And so it is with hari kari cosmetic surgery. As long as people want to undergo the procedure in order to change their appearance, then there will always be surgeons and centers available to accommodate them. It will only stop when people, through their own individual decision-making process, decide to follow a different path.

20

Weight Loss Drugs—Forcing a Healthy System to Malfunction

In no other area has big Pharma encountered the number of disasters that has plagued it in the weight loss arena. Amphetamines caused addiction; digitalis and diuretics directly caused deaths; Aminorex resulted in pulmonary hypertension; fenfluramine and phentermine (the so-called Fen/Phen drugs) resulted in heart valve insufficiency; and Sibutramine (Reductil/Meridia) has been banned due to the high level of heart and other problems among people who have been taking it.

All these drugs were all put on the market with great fanfare, only to be pulled when their disastrous side effects were uncovered.[1] At the time of this writing, the only drug that is still FDA approved for long-term use is Orlistat (Xenical/Alli).

Why? Why have diet drugs produced such lethal, catastrophic results while in other areas, the pharmaceutical industry has been enormously successful in treating and sometimes curing many serious problems? The reason is that diet drugs are designed to do something fundamentally different from all other pharmaceutical products.

Other pharmaceutical products either help the body fight off outside invasions from viruses or bacteria, or they try to correct the problems associated with malfunctioning systems. If you have heart disease, something in your heart is malfunctioning and there are drugs that can help correct that. Similarly, if you have hypertension, high cholesterol, or diabetes, there are organs or systems that are not functioning properly in your body and there are drugs that are designed to fix that.

Diet drugs are totally different. They are designed to make a perfectly healthy system malfunction. When your food energy intake exceeds the energy that you expend, the body stores that extra energy as fat. This is exactly and precisely what it is supposed to do. It is functioning normally.

In order for a diet drug to work, it must make your fat storage system malfunction. It has to make it stop working the way it is supposed to work. And when you try to make a person's basic survival system malfunction, you have to use a pretty massive sledge-hammer, and there has been untold collateral damage.

Even Orlistat (marketed as the prescription drug Xenical by Roche pharmaceuticals or as an over-the-counter product called Alli by GlaxoSmithKline), the only long-term use drug still on the market, is a malfunction-inducing drug. It forces your intestinal system to malfunction by interfering with its fat absorption mechanism. Essentially, it forces your body to go on a diet, not by limiting what you eat, but by derailing your digestive system so it can't properly process everything you eat.

Orlistat also has some unpleasant side effects including "steatorrhea (oily, loose stools with excessive flatus due to unabsorbed fats reaching the large intestine), fecal incontinence [euphemistically referred to as anal leakage] and frequent or urgent bowel movements."[2]

Orlistat also demands a meticulous adherence to certain protocols. It requires that you take one pill with each meal and carefully limit your fat intake.

Although Orlistat is still on the market, the FDA is currently investigating thirty-two reports of serious liver injury, including six cases of liver failure, in patients using Orlistat.[3] And it has been implicated in hospitalizations for kidney problems.[4]

A lot of people consider using weight loss pills because they have "tried to diet before and it hasn't worked." But before you make that assumption, go back and look at your responses to the little quiz in Chapter 11.

Look at how many pounds you have lost over the years. Is it really that you don't know how to diet and lose weight or is it that you are a very proficient dieter, but you always put the pounds back on? If you really feel you need to lose weight and you have had success in dieting in the past, but have always put the weight back on, forget pills. You don't need them.

Weight loss pills aren't magical. They do the same thing that a diet does, which is to create a calorie deficit. You already know how to do that without pills. The issue is not getting the weight off. It is keeping the weight off. And Orlistat (Xenical/Alli) won't do that. It will plateau after a while and then you will slowly start to regain the weight (assuming you are not following a fitness program) even if you keep taking the pills.[5,6] Of course, the pharmaceutical companies marketing this drug want you to stay on the medication forever. But when you plateau, it's done all it can for you.

So if you want to lose weight, and you've had success in losing weight before but not in keeping it off, then go back and lose weight until you plateau. Then depend on your 10,000 steps a day fitness program to keep it off. If you've lost enough in your first shot, then just stay where you are. If you decide you need to lose more, just rinse and repeat until you are satisfied with your weight.

Of course, that has not stopped big Pharma, since there is a massive pot of gold at the end of the rainbow for anyone who can come up with a truly effective and truly safe diet drug. So you can be sure they'll be baaack.

21

Weight Loss Programs

There is a huge variety of weight loss programs available.

For-profit programs without medical supervision include Weight Watchers, Jenny Craig (owned by Nestlé), and LA Weight Loss. Medically supervised programs include OPTIFAST (which is owned by Novartis pharmaceuticals), Health Management Resources, and Medifast/Take Shape for Life. There are also product-only programs such as Slim Fast and endless other options.

The two biggest nonprofit programs are Overeaters Anonymous and TOPS (Take off Pounds Sensibly).

Overeaters Anonymous operates on the same twelve-step principles as does Alcoholics Anonymous and is completely free. The TOPS model is closer to that of Weight Watchers with weekly group meetings and weigh-ins. It has a small initial registration fee and a five dollar a month ongoing fee to cover the organization's costs.

A study in 2005 looked at the major programs to see how they worked and how much they cost.[1] The result was that it was really hard to tell how well the programs worked in comparison to each other because so much depends on personal adherence to the program. Basically, they all work, sort of, if you adhere to them.

Costs are another story. They range from free or practically free for Overeaters Anonymous and TOPS, up to thousands of dollars for some programs. Before signing on for any program, make absolutely sure that you know exactly what all the costs are. Costs can include an initial membership fee, required medical evaluation, weekly or monthly fees, required purchase of materials, and required purchase of full or partial meal replacements.

So yes, you can use these programs to take it off. Surprise, you already knew that. The key question as always is, can you keep it off? In fact, there is a study titled "Three-year follow-up of participants in a commercial weight-loss program. Can you keep it off?" Answer: "The frequency of exercise after the diet program was the strongest predictor of weight loss maintenance."[2] Surprise!

The only way you can keep it off is to be fit. But is keeping it off in the long-term business interest of these companies? The business models of weight loss programs require that they succeed short term. They must succeed in providing short-term weight loss so that they have a reputation for success and can attract new and repeat customers.

But what about the long term? If they succeeded in providing long-term weight loss, would they be able to stay in business? The problem is that if they succeeded in providing long-term weight loss, people who wanted to lose weight would do so and they would keep the weight off. Thus, they would be lost as customers. Eventually, everyone would be at the weight they preferred and these programs would go out of business.

Now of course, just about every weight loss program out there always says "diet and exercise, diet and exercise, diet and exercise." But although some people like exercise or find it fulfilling or satisfying, most people don't.

Pushing exercise—instead of a 10,000 step walking program that people really will do—is doomed to failure since most people don't like exercise and therefore won't exercise.

So if you aren't going to start and maintain a 10,000 step fitness walking program (or use some other physical activity to burn that extra 2,000 extra calories a week), **DON'T SIGN UP FOR THESE PROGRAMS. IN FACT, DON'T DIET AT ALL.**

Without fitness, you are practically guaranteed to put the weight back on again. And as you diet and put it back on, and diet and put it back on, and diet and put it back on, you'll ultimately convince your body that famines are a frequent event and that it has to raise your set point to keep you safe. As a result, you'll end up weighing more than you did when you started.

22

Diet Books—6' 6" Long

I live in a small suburban town. Its population is just under 8,000. We have a nice little library. The other day I stopped in the library and went to the section on diet books. I brought a tape measure with me. The diet book section was 6' 6" long. I counted 71 diet books.

If you go to Amazon, and type in "diet books," it will give you thousands of results.

There are psychology diet books (Joy, Shangri-la, Good Mood, Instinct). There are place diet books (Wall Street, Duke University). There are celebrity diet books (Deepak Chopra, Schwarzenegger,

Suzanne Somers). There are beach diet books (South Beach, Muscle Beach, Nude Beach). There are time diet books (12 Seconds, 17 days, 75 years). There are what you eat diet books (Fiber, Protein, Tulip Petals, Fat, Carbs). The list is endless.

And you know what? The great majority of them cut your calories in one way or another. If you decide to follow one of them (and please make sure you eat a balanced diet and stay away from the really weird ones—we don't recommend the root beer and kimchi diet), you will lose weight. Surprise! You already knew that.

But the same issue rears its ugly head. Can you keep it off? And you already know the answer to that. So I'm going to simply repeat what I said in the last chapter.

The only way you can keep it off is to be fit. If you aren't going to start and maintain a 10,000 step fitness walking program (or use some other physical activity to burn 2,000 extra calories a week) **DON'T FOLLOW ANY OF THESE DIET PLANS. IN FACT, DON'T DIET AT ALL.**

Without fitness, you are practically guaranteed to put the weight back on again. And as you diet and put it back on, and diet and put it back on, and diet and put it back on, you'll ultimately convince your body that famines are a frequent event and that it has to raise your set point to keep you safe. As a result, you'll end up weighing more than you did when you started.

23

The Magic, Glowing Amberonium-Zircrohmic Weight Loss Pentagon

Dear Mom,

I am so excited I can hardly sit still to write this. I get to tell you a great big "I told you so." It works. It really, really works and we have proven it. I know that you laughed at my Magic, Glowing Amberonium-Zircrohmic Weight Loss Pentagon, despite the fact that we tested it on dogs and they lost weight and then on pigs and they lost weight—and I can tell you that the farmers who owned the pigs weren't thrilled.

And then we put it on the market. Some people bought it and a few positive testimonials came in, but you know, it just wasn't enough. No one really believed that it could work.

But then I got lucky. At a weight loss conference I had the great fortune to meet Dr. I. M. Skeptical, PhD, and Dr. B.S. Sniffer, PhD. At first, the conversation was a bit rocky. They growled at me for selling junk and told me I shouldn't be such a scam artist. But I handed each of them ten Magic, Glowing Amberonium-Zircrohmic Weight Loss Pentagons and said "Prove me wrong, if you can."

Well. That was a challenge they could not pass up. They tested it on twenty people. To their incredible amazement, seventeen people lost a pound a week over ten weeks and the other three lost three quarters of a pound a week.

Based on that, they agreed to recruit 1,000 volunteers and do a randomized, double-blind research study. I supplied them with 500 real full-size Pentagons and 500 identical looking non-magic full-size pentagons.

The experimental results are now in. The 500 people who got the non-magic pentagons didn't lose any weight at all. But 85 percent of the people who wore the real Magic, Glowing Amberonium-Zircrohmic Weight Loss Pentagons lost a pound a week over twenty weeks and the rest lost three-quarters of a pound a week.

Then, in the next step of the experiment, the 500 people who lost weight were again randomly split into two groups. Two hundred fifty were given real, half-size Magic, Glowing Amberonium-Zircrohmic Weight Maintenance Pentagons and the other 250 were given fake weight maintenance pentagons.

They then followed them for a full year. The people with the real half-size maintenance Magic, Glowing Amberonium-Zircrohmic Weight Maintenance Pentagons kept the weight off and didn't put a pound back on. The people who were given the fake weight maintenance pentagons put most of the weight that they had lost back on again.

They have now written up the results of their experiment and it will be published in the *New England Journal of Medicine* next week. And Mom, I'm going to be a bazillion, gazillionaire.

Your Loving Son

Just think. If you truly invented something that really worked, just like the Magic, Glowing Amberonium-Zircrohmic Weight Loss Pentagon, the first thing that you would do would be to get a hold of Dr. I. M. Skeptical, PhD, and Dr. B.S. Sniffer, PhD and have them test it. Then they would write it up, it would be published in a peer-reviewed journal, and everybody would know that it worked and you would be a bazillion, gazillionaire.

So what about all the magic miracle weight-loss products sold on the Internet and in infomercials. Do they work? It's real simple. **SHOW ME THE**

RESEARCH. Not the research you claimed to do on fifteen people. And not the research done by "a respected researcher" except that you don't mention that respected researcher's name and don't give us the peer-reviewed journal article in which the results were published. Show me the real research.

Let's look at some of the Magic, Glowing Amberonium-Zircrohmic weight loss products on the market.

1. Magic Spot Reducers

Sorry, that's not how the body works. If you use an ab machine or similar contraption, you'll do great things for your abs, but you won't reduce the fat that surrounds those muscles.

> But what about bodybuilders? They work all those muscles and they get really ripped. So spot reducing must work.

Bodybuilding has to be one of the world's weirdest sports. When bodybuilders are building muscle, they need to eat 4,000 to 5,000 calories a day, that's how hard they're working. But bodybuilding goes in phases. First, there's the muscle building phase and then there's the show phase. During the show phase, bodybuilders go on freakishly low calorie diets, sometimes less than 1,000 calories a day. They burn off every ounce of fat so that all that is left is muscle.

If you use an ab machine or do any weight lifting, the body will recruit energy evenly from across your body in the same way as it would if you were walking or jumping rope or doing anything else. It does not recruit energy from the specific spots where you are working your muscles.

If you have any doubts, look at a short YouTube video showing Antonio Krastev setting a world record of 475 pounds in the snatch competition.[1] The snatch requires incredible strength in the legs, abdomen, chest, and arms. As you'll see, Mr. Krastev doesn't look anything like a Mr. Universe, even though he is probably stronger than any bodybuilder who ever lived.

2. Magic Diet Food

Slimee Dimee Citrus Micro Nutrient Activated Tap Water ($19.95 per 12 oz. bottle). Super Thin Caramel Flavored Sawdust Power Bar ($14.95 each).

3. Magic Diet Pills—Over-the-counter or from the Internet

Don't even think about it. For example, in July of 2010, the Food and Drug Administration recalled something called Joyful Slim Herb Supplement when a lab analysis found that it contained desmethyl sibutramine. That's right, the same sibutramine that has been banned in the U.S. and Europe because it causes heart problems.[2]

And that is just the tip of the iceberg. A study of eighty-one over-the-counter products determined that 73 percent contained sibutramine, as well as a host of other nasty things, including the banned drug Fenfluramine.[3]

Bottom line—stay away from this stuff. You have absolutely no idea what is in these things and you have no reliable way of finding out.

4. Magic Cleanses

Do you need a purge? You absolutely do if your nuclearic toxin levels have reached bivalent stratification levels. And they almost certainly have if you do things like eat food. Magic Organic Purges, Inc. has your answer. For just $72.50 a day, delivered straight from our organic juicer to your doorstep, you get the healthful, nutritious deep cleanse that your body craves.

> "I don't know. I read that a respected scientist thinks that cleansing is dangerous. That makes me a little worried."[4]

Don't listen to him. He's a dork.

> "Okay, but did you at least run it by Dr. I. M. Skeptical, PhD, and Dr. B.S. Sniffer, PhD?"

Oh, come on. They're such fuddy duddys. They wouldn't know a good thing if it came up and bit them in the butt. I hate to say this, but I have never seen such a severe case of toxin-induced skepticitis. Your out-of-control negativity is totally symptomatic. You really just have to trust us. We are Magic Organic Purges, Inc. We love you and we are here to help you.

Now just tell me again, what was the expiration date on your credit card?

5. Magic "I lost 23 pounds in three weeks" Diets

Let's do a hypothetical thought experiment. Imagine that you were shipwrecked on a desert island for seven days with plenty of water but no food. And then, exactly seven days after you washed up on the island, a rescue boat finds you. You are saved and live happily ever after.

How much weight did you lose during those seven days? First, let's assume that your breakeven point is 1,750 calories (just to make the math easier). That is, on a normal day your body uses 1,750 calories of energy, so that if you eat exactly that many calories, you will neither gain or lose weight.

A pound of fat contains about 3,500 calories. Given that your breakeven is 1,750, you lost three and a half pounds during those seven days (7 x 1,750 ÷ 3,500 = 3.5). Anything more would just be water loss, but since you had plenty of water, you just lost 3.5 pounds.

So how could anyone lose twenty-three pounds in three weeks? If you really ate nothing whatsoever for three weeks, you would lose 10.5 pounds. To lose twenty-three pounds, you would also have to have lost 12.5 pounds of water, that is if you were still alive at the end the three weeks.

6. Magic Corset Products

Corset-type things that tighten you up to make you look thinner. Compression shapers, body shapers, hip squeezers, you name it. And of course, they all work just great—until you have to breathe.

PART
V

How the Weight Loss Industry Tricked
Us into Believing That Fat Is a Disease
and What We Can Do about It

24

The Obesity Researchaganda Machine Just Keeps Going and Going and Going

At the beginning of this book, I promised you that it would be WOSWAK free. In other words, that there wouldn't be a lot of warmed over stuff that you already knew. And I suspect that most people are not really aware of all or most of the research that we have highlighted here. In one sense, that's good. But looked at another way, it's really appalling.

A lot of the research is not all that new. Dr. Wei's study, proving that fitness overcomes any negative health consequences attributed to weight, was

published in 1999. Dr. Pavlou's study showing that
fitness prevented weight regain after dieting was
published all the way back in 1989. So how come everyone doesn't have this information right at their
fingertips?

The answer, unfortunately, is that the Weight
Loss Industry really, really doesn't want you to know
about it. As we said, fitness is the most serious threat
facing the profitability of the Weight Loss Industry.

Now obviously, they can't suppress the information, so what they do is simply drown it in a sea of
Obesity Epidemic researchaganda (researchaganda
= research used as marketing propaganda).

We live in a 24/7 news cycle, Twitter feeding, Facebook posting, information overload universe. What
gets repeated the most gets remembered. And what
gets repeated the most is Obesity Epidemic, Obesity
Epidemic, Obesity Epidemic. It drowns out everything
else, in part because there's so much of it, and in part
because almost nobody is standing up to counter it.

Over just a few months time the following headlines and text appeared:

***Obesity Care May Cost Twice Previous Esti-
mates:*** "Nearly 17 percent of US medical costs
can be blamed on obesity."[1]

***Nearly 30 percent of Americans Likely to Have
Diabetes by 2050:*** "People are becoming fatter.
Overweight/obesity are key risk factors for dia-
betes type 2."[2]

UnitedHealth Predicts $3.4 Trillion Diabetes Decade[3]

Life Expectancy for Today's Youth Cut Short by Obesity: "For the first time in history, the next generation will not live longer, or even as long, as their parents."[4]

Cost of Obesity Approaching $300 Billion a Year[5]

Obesity Weighs down Cities' Budgets. Trimming Obesity Would Save US Cities Millions in Healthcare Costs, Study Finds: "Trimming high obesity rates in the nation's most overweight cities could help local governments save more than $32 billion annually nationwide...."[6]

Why Are Men Getting So Tubby? "Last week, Oxford University scientists reported that the average man is more than a stone heavier—17 pounds—than 20 years ago."[7]

Bariatric Surgery Cuts Pounds, and Adds Years: "Obese individuals may add years to their lives by drastically cutting pounds with bariatric surgery."[8]

Study: Being Even a Little Fat a Health Risk: "Having a little extra meat on your bones—if that meat happens to be fat—is harmful, not beneficial."[9]

Global Obesity Rates Are Doubling: New World-wide Study: "Obesity is a chronic metabolic disease in which excess body fat has accumulated to the extent that it may have detrimental effect on human life expectancy, leading to multiple health problems."[10]

Notice that all these stories reported on research studies that had just been published.

Who are the people who conduct this kind of research? No, for the most part they aren't flacks bought and paid for by the Weight Loss Industry, even though it is true that many studies are funded by Weight Loss Industry companies, some researchers have conflicts of interest because they give paid speeches at Weight Loss Industry conferences, and some do consulting for companies in the Weight Loss Industry.

However, on the whole, they are usually well meaning researchers. So why do they do it?

Perhaps because it's popular and in fashion. And of course, there is lots of funding available for obesity studies. Maybe they have simply bought into the fat is bad mythos created by the Weight Loss Industry. And it's also conceivable that some of them are simply fatistas. That is they have a deep-seated, visceral negative reaction to how heavy people look, and the very idea that heavy people could be fit and perfectly healthy simply may not compute for them.

But regardless of the reasons, they churn out study after study that mainly function as marketing and branding tools for the Weight Loss Industry.

In fact, the words obesity and obesity epidemic might just as well be registered trademarks of the Weight Loss Industry (of course, then every time you wrote those words, you would have to use the trademark symbol ® and they would have to be written like this—Obesity® or Obesity Epidemic®).

They serve the same function for the Weight Loss Industry that "Got Milk?"® serves for the California Milk Processor Board and "You Deserve a Break Today"® serves for McDonald's.

And of course, the media laps it up. The media lives for dire warnings of impending catastrophe and the Obesity Epidemic is a gift that keeps on giving, and giving, and giving.

And so one hand continuously feeds the other. The researchers produce the researchaganda, the media feeds on it, and as a result, we get a continuous diet of Obesity Epidemic researchaganda. And everybody assumes that, because it's repeated so often, it simply must be true.

So how do you counter that? We will get into how that can be done in a moment, but first I think it would be worthwhile to review briefly the history of how we got to this place. If you find history bo-o-o-r-i-n-g, just go ahead and skip down to Chapter 27, Derailing Obesity Epidemic Researchaganda—The Media Response Team.

25

Celebrating "Obesity Epidemic" Day

Each year on March 10, the Weight Loss Industry quietly celebrates "Obesity Epidemic" Day, commemorating the publication on March 10, 2004 of a monumental piece of researchaganda with the innocuous sounding title "Actual Causes of Death in the United States, 2000."[1]

The publication of this paper was the culmination of many years of intensive efforts by the Weight Loss Industry to create the Obesity Epidemic and define fat as a disease.[2] It constitutes one of the most incredibly successful (and destructive) special interest lobbying coup d'états ever recorded.

Here is what happened. Up until about 1995, it was pretty much accepted that the healthiest weight was somewhere in the BMI 23 to 27 range. A huge study of 1.7 million people in Norway showed that, for the general population, the longest life expectancy was BMI 21–27 for men and BMI 23–27 for women.[3]

However, by 1995, the International Obesity Task Force (IOTF), an industry trade group funded primarily by Hoffman LaRoche and Abbott Laboratories (makers of the weight loss drugs Xenical and Meridia [now banned due to heart problems] respectively), had taken control of the decision-making process of the World Health Organization when it came to defining what was overweight.

The 1995 World Health Organization report, written primarily by IOTF, created three categories. Below BMI 25 was labeled "Normal." BMI 25 to 30 was labeled "Overweight" and above the BMI 30 was labeled "Obese." (IOTF probably wanted to classify these last two as "Abnormal" and "Freakishly Abnormal," but I guess they concluded that even they couldn't get away with that.)[4]

The next step was the takeover of the NIH (National Institutes of Health) through its Obesity Task Force. Seven of the nine members of the task force were, believe it or not, directors of weight loss clinics. Who better to expand the definition of obesity?

They issued a report in June of 1998 lowering the standards for obesity and overweight to conform to those in the hijacked World Health Organization report. (One of the two members of the task force, who were not part of the Weight Loss Industry, was asked why they accepted the World Health Organization definitions when the evidence pointed in the opposite direction. She is reported to have replied that they were "pressured to make the standards conform" to the World Health Organization's hijacked report.[5])

The final step in the Weight Loss Industry's coup d'état was the publication on March 10, 2004 in the *Journal of the American Medical Association* of "Actual Causes of Death in the United States, 2000" which claimed (falsely as it turned out) that obesity was responsible for 400,000 deaths a year in the United States. The report received massive media attention[6], and thus was born the Obesity Epidemic.

The implications for the Weight Loss Industry were huge. Prior to this, the main reason people sought out the services of the Weight Loss Industry was because they wished to change their appearance.

Now the Weight Loss Industry's decade-long campaign to have fat falsely branded as a disease had come to fruition and the government had certified that carrying extra weight was a serious health problem. With the credibility of the government behind them, the Weight Loss Industry could now not only claim that they would make you look different, but they could now assert that they would also save your life. This obviously created substantial increased demand for their services.

Up until the publication of the **Obesity = 400,000 Deaths Panic Panic** researchaganda report in 2004, weight was essentially an issue of aesthetics.

With the publication of that report, even though it was quickly debunked, the perception that fat was a disease became embedded in the public psyche, a perception that is repeatedly reinforced by government health bureaucrats and everybody in the Weight Loss Industry.

26

Something Is Very Rotten in Denmark

It turns out that this **Obesity = 400,000 Deaths Panic Panic** researchaganda report was written, not by the CDC's top experts in the field, but by the CDC director Julie Gerberding, who has no particular expertise in the subject, and by other researchers in her office.[1]

Needless to say, Gerberding trumpeted the report a few days later when she went to Congress to beg for more money for her agency's budget.

But it didn't take long for the "you know what" to hit the fan. In early May, *Science Magazine* reported that epidemiologists at the CDC and the National Institutes of Health had serious concerns about the report's data and the methodology. (The culture of fear within the agencies was so strong that these researchers refused to give their names because, as one of them said, "I don't want to lose my job.")[2]

The report was such a mess that even *The Wall Street Journal*, that dedicated champion of all things business and fierce foe of all things governmental and regulatory, smelled a rat. It reported that the CDC's experts on the subject had warned about problems with the **Obesity = 400,000 Deaths Panic Panic** report but were ignored. It was also reported that Dr. Terry Pechacek, Associate Director for Science in the CDC's Office on Smoking and Health stated that "I would never have cleared this paper if I had been given the opportunity to provide a formal review."[3]

Eventually, Congress got into the act and demanded that the Government Accountability Office conduct an investigation. A year later the CDC published a summary of the investigation admitting "significant limitations" to the **Obesity = 400,000 Deaths Panic Panic** report. They refused, however, to release the full investigative report.

It was only when a Freedom of Information Act demand was filed that the full investigative report was released. Needless to say, it fully exposed the con game in the **Obesity = 400,000 Deaths Panic Panic** report.[4]

Of course, the whole discussion is about the wrong issue. Studies continue to be produced on a regular basis arguing which BMI group has the lowest death rate, but since they don't separate their study popu-lations between fit and unfit, the whole exercise is meaningless. Here's why.

Let's say you did a study that examined two groups of people. In one group you had 10,000 peo-ple in the so-called "normal" BMI level of 25 or less. In the other group you had 10,000 people in the so-called "obese" BMI level of 30 or more.

Now let's imagine two sets of possibilities for this study. With the first possibility, all the people in the "normal" group are fit and all the people in the "obese" group are unfit. What you would find is that the "obese" group had an all-cause mortality rate that was three times greater than the "normal" group.

In the second possibility, all the people in the "normal" group are unfit and all the people in the "obese" group are fit. Now what you would find would be that the people in the "obese" group had just half the all-cause mortality rate of the people in the "nor-mal" group.

So as you can see, studies that don't differentiate between the fitness of the people being studied pro-duce garbage results. They are basically meaningless.

However, they're just exactly the kind of resear-chaganda that the Weight Loss Industry loves, be-cause it keeps the discussion going around the issue of how much fat is too much, while the underlying as-sumption that fat is a disease never gets questioned.

27

Derailing Obesity Epidemic Researchaganda: The Media Response Team

So how do we derail the Weight Loss Industry's researchaganda message that has been so successfully ingrained into the public psyche? We derail it with a huge volume of messages that expose the researchaganda for what it is and tell the true story. If enough people get involved in a mass truthaganda movement, we can begin to change the public's perception.

And how do we produce this huge volume of messages? Well, that's where you can play a critical role. I can get on the phone or blog or do interviews from morning until night and hardly dent the surface. But if, when a piece of researchaganda comes out, you get on the phone with people you know, or put something in your blog if you have one, or tweet, or post something on your Facebook page, then we will start to have an impact.

Even better, I'd like to suggest that you consider going public and do some media interviews. Now before you yell at me that you've never done an interview, and you don't know any reporters, and who would want to listen to you anyway, let me tell you why you absolutely have the right stuff to do this.

Let's start with why the media would want to listen to you. Remember, we said that the media loves stories about dire warnings of impending catastrophe. In fact, there's only one thing that they love better and that's controversy. Now they'll have both in one. You'll be responding to a researchaganda study—"dire warning"—with a contrary point of view—"controversy."

You'll also be adding something else that they really lap up. The media likes nothing better than to flesh out any story with a human interest point of view. That's you. You aren't an industry. You're a private citizen who was concerned enough to call them to set the record straight. That's practically a story in itself.

And finally, the media wants to deal with experts. What's an expert? An expert is someone with deep knowledge. You've gotten this far in the book so you now have general deep knowledge and you'll also have specific knowledge (which we will share with you in advance) about the researchaganda piece that you will be commenting on.

So you have the perfect recipe for the media: dire warnings, controversy, human interest, and expertise.

But you don't know anybody in the media, right? Well, maybe you actually do. But let's assume you don't, so how do you find them? There are two ways.

The first is through networking. Do you have any friends who work in or have experience with any aspect of media? Do any of your friends' friends work in or have any experience with any aspect of media? You're almost sure to find somebody. After all, if you have twenty friends or acquaintances, and each of them have twenty friends or acquaintances, then you have immediate access to 400 people at least.

Connect with the ones you find who have media expertise, tell them what you're thinking of doing, and ask for some mentoring and advice. You'll be amazed at what you'll get, and then you're off and running.

The second way is to pay attention to which reporters do health-related stories in your local newspaper or on your local radio station (or TV station if you would like to get on camera). Then, when a new study comes out, you can call the newspaper or radio station and ask to speak with that person. Just say to the reporter, or whoever picks up the phone, "There's a new study out claiming that 142% of the population will die of obesity within the next six months. Is anybody doing a story on that? If so, I'd like to share with them a really interesting contrary point of view."

Okay, so now you have a reporter on the phone. How do you do a good interview? A good interview requires three things. First, you need to be aware that reporters are always in a mad rush. They have deadlines and lots of people to interview, so they really appreciate it when you are quick and to the point.

Second, be yourself and know your stuff. Being authentic and having accurate information are the keys to your credibility.

Third, have three key points you want to make. Why just three, when there are thirty-seven really important things that you might want to say? Because at best, you're only going to get three quotes into the story. If you let the reporter or editor choose which of your thirty-seven points they're going to use, they probably won't choose the most important ones or the ones you want them to use. If you just give them three and keep restating them in different ways, guess what, those are the ones they're going to use.

How will you know your stuff, have accurate information, and be able to develop those three key points? Whenever a study comes out, we will read it, analyze it, and put it up on the GreatFatFraud.com Media Response Team page. It will describe the study and what's wrong with it, and where appropriate, it will give you links to the really good studies that tell the true story and will show you how to walk a reporter through those studies to get to the key information quickly.

Working with reporters is really about building relationships. You start slowly, get to know a couple of the reporters, build your credibility with authenticity and accurate information, and pretty soon, they'll be calling you for a response before you call them.

If you'd really rather not do interviews, you can still tweet about the study and your response to it, post something on a Facebook page, or otherwise connect through your social media network. And of course, you can do both interviews and social media networking if you like.

So please, consider being part of the Media Response Team. Together we can derail the Weight Loss's researchaganda Obesity Epidemic machine and really make a change in public perception.

PART
VI

Putting It All Together

28

Where Are the Recipes?

That's it? We're done?

That's it. We're done.

But where are the fifty-five pages of recipes for delicious, nutritious, easy-to-prepare meals?

There are a bazillion recipes on the Internet. Anything you want is there. You certainly don't need more recipes here, and anyway, I am a lousy chef.

But what about the one-week fitness plan, and the thirteen-week plan, and the fifty-two week plan and the seventy-five-year plan?

You don't need those plans. Just listen to your body. Any plan I could put here would be wrong for you. It would tell you to either go too fast or go too slow. Your body is unique. It doesn't matter if it takes you six months or two years to get to 10,000 steps. All that matters is that you get there and that you feel comfortable doing it.

Just identify your baseline, add 500 steps a day, and stay there until that's really, really comfortable, then add 500 more and keep going till eventually you get to 10,000. Don't rush, just listen to your body.

So you can just summarize this whole book in a single paragraph?

Walk 10,000 steps a day and you will eliminate any negative health consequences associated with weight. Walk 10,000 steps a day and you won't gain weight. Walk 10,000 steps a day and if you decide to diet and lose weight, you will be able to keep it off. And then, tell everyone else about it, so they will do it too.

That's it?

That's it.

But it's so simple.

Absolutely. Enjoy.

PART
VII

Endnotes and More Detail on the
Science Underlying This Book

29

Introduction

In developing this book, one of the things that we struggled with (my editors and I) was what level of detail should be in the book itself and which details should be reserved for the endnotes section.

In the book, we wanted to provide only those details that were absolutely necessary for a clear understanding of the science. Sometimes we provided a lot of detail for the key studies. In other cases, we've simply alluded to studies without saying much about them.

In this section, we've tried to fill in those blanks and provide more detail on the science that underlies everything in this book. You don't have to read this endnote section if you are not interested, because everything you absolutely need to know is in the book. But if you're curious and want to know more, it's here.

This section also provides the detailed citation for each study noted in the book, and where an abstract of the study or the whole study itself is available online; we have provided the URL so that you can download it. We've also tried to provide a little bit of a road map for each study to make it easier to find the key information, should you decide to download it.

Links to all the studies, abstracts, and articles that are available for download can be found at www. greatfatfraud.com on the "Book Reference Links" page.

30

Endnotes and More Details on the Science Underlying This Book

Chapter 3: Fitlessness

1. Much of the justification for the Obesity Epidemic myth comes from large population studies that look only at weight and death rates. As we'll see in Chapter 4, these kinds of studies produce false results because they omit the key determining variable. However, it's important to know a little bit about this kind of study.

    A good example of this kind of study is "BMI and Mortality: Results from a National Longitudinal Study of Canadian Adults" (*Obesity* 2009, 18:214–218) by Orpana1, H., Berthelot, J.,Kaplan, M. et al. The full study is available at (http://www .nature.com/oby/journal/v18/n1/pdf/oby2009191a.pdf). Go to the "Book References Links" page at www.greatfatfraud .com for a direct link to the study.

    This study, like so many others in its category, accepts the false premise that being heavy, in and of itself, increases the risk of mortality. The study simply chimes in on the ongoing argument over how much weight is okay and how much is dangerous.

    I am going to go into quite a bit of detail on this study. The reason is that many of the terms and approaches used here are used in the other studies the book will reference. Therefore, this will be something of a primer on how to read these studies in general.

    The heart of this study is Table 3 on page 217. (Note that in academic journals, page numbering is by volume. Journals publish one or two volumes per year. The first page of the January issue will be page 1 and a paper published in May might start on page 731.)

Table 3 shows nine categories of BMI starting with 18.5, which is dangerously underweight [see the boxed text at the end of this endnote for more information on BMI]. The next column under the letter "n" shows the number of people in each category in the study and to the right of that, the percent that that makes up of the total study. In the total study, there were 286 participants who were under BMI 18.5 and they made up 2 percent of the total population of the study.

Finally, and this is the meat of the whole article, is a column titled Adjusted RR (95 percent Confidence Interval). "RR" stands for the group's average relative risk of death compared to the reference group (a term we'll meet often in scientific studies) and the confidence interval shows the distribution of the results.

And just exactly what does the above paragraph of convoluted gobbledygook mean? Well, when scientists do a study, they're generally measuring things. To measure things they need a reference point. The generally accepted convention in these kinds of studies is to choose BMI 25, the so-called "normal" weight, as the reference point and assign it a value of 1.0. Then you measure all the other groups and see whether their rate of death is higher or lower than the reference group.

If you go up to the first line, you'll see that the average rate of death for those whose weight is under BMI 18.5 is 1.89, which means that the rate of death for this group is fully 89 percent higher than that of the reference group. The 1.89 figure is an average and so the study gives you the distribution at the 95 percent confidence interval. What this means is that most of the 286 people in this group had rates of death that fell between 36 percent higher than the reference group and 164 percent higher than the reference group. Clearly being this underweight is very dangerous indeed.

As you look down the table, you see something fascinating. The two groups in the so-called "overweight" group have death rates that are below the BMI 25—the so-called "normal"—group. Even in the next two groups, which cover BMI 30 to 35, and which the Weight Loss Industry labels as "obese," we see that the rates of death are just a little above and just a little bit below those of the so-called "normal" group. It's only when we get into the BMI above 35 group that we see death rates starting to climb.

However, this still does not demonstrate that being that heavy is dangerous since the key variable that would tell us what is really going on is not part of the study.

About BMI

Most studies on weight, including this one, classify weight using the BMI scale. You can find a BMI table in Appendix 1. Basically, the table relates height to weight and produces a number. The table itself is nonjudgmental. It is simply a constructed number. The advantage of such a table is that it recognizes that the taller people are, the more they're likely to weigh. It is reasonably internally consistent, which means that it measures what it says it measures, unless you happen to be a weightlifter or are otherwise very muscular, in which case it will throw it off since muscle is a bit heavier than other tissue.

Although some people have complained about the BMI scale, particularly because of the muscle weight issue for bodybuilders, it more or less measures what it says it measures. The problem is how the scale has been used to define "good" and "bad" levels of weight.

To make a long story short (and we will go into this in more detail in Part V), the Weight Loss Industry hijacked a committee of the World Health Organization and got it to label people who were BMI 25 to 30 as overweight and people who were BMI 30 and above as obese. Shortly thereafter, the health bureaucracy in the U.S. bought into these definitions.

The flies in this ointment are twofold. First, a lot of studies have shown that when you look at the general population, the lowest death rates occur in the so-called "overweight" BMI 25 to 30 group. The Canadian study is a good example of this.

Second, it turns out that weight is not really relevant when it comes to all-cause mortality and that it really is another variable that drives mortality rates.

2. Smith E. "Report on the Sanitary Condition of Tailors in London," as reported in *Report of the Medical Officer*, London, The Privy Council, 1864:416–430 as reported in Domhnall MacAuley, A History of Physical Activity, Health and Medicine. *J. of the Royal Society of Med.* 1994; 87, 32–35. (http://www.ncbi.nlm.nih.gov/pmc/articles/PMC1294279 /pdf/jrsocmed00089-0044.pdf)

This is a nice little review of the thinking about the relationship between physical activity and health going all the way back to ancient times. The discussion of the tailors study is on page 34.

3. Morris JN, Heady JA, Raffle PAB, et al. "Coronary heart disease and the physical activity of work." *Lancet* 1953; 2: 1053–1057, 1111–1120. Unfortunately, this study is not available online.

The study included approximately 31,000 men ages thirty-five to sixty-four. The study found that the conductors, who were extremely active and had to climb up and down the stairs of the double-decker buses all day, had a rate of heart attacks and of fatal heart attacks that was half that of the more sedentary drivers. (Table III, page 1055)

When he looked at the postal workers, he found that the postmen who delivered the mail had a rate of coronary heart disease that was 50 percent of the postal workers who were mostly sedentary, such as those working the telephones and civil-service executives. He also included a middle group that had an intermediate amount of physical activity, such as people who worked the counter, postal supervisors, and higher-grade postmen. He found that this middle group had rates of heart disease that was precisely in the middle of the other two groups. (Table VI, page 1056)

An excellent and very readable review of Jeremy Morris' work can be found in Paffenbarger RS Jr, Blair SN, Lee IM. "A history of physical activity, cardiovascular health and longevity: the scientific contributions of Jeremy N Morris." *Int J Epidemiol.* 2001;30:1184–1192. (http://ije.oxfordjournals .org/content/30/5/1184.full.pdf+html)

4. Blair, S, Kohl, H, Paffenbarger, R, et al. "Physical Fitness and All-Cause Mortality, A Prospective Study of Healthy Men and Women." *JAMA* 1989; 262:2395–2401 (http://jama.ama-assn.org/content/262/17/2395.full.pdf+html)

What makes this study special is that it was the first really large-scale study of the relationship between ***measured*** fitness and all-cause mortality. Prior studies had focused primarily on physical activities as reported in questionnaires filled out by participants. Unfortunately, physical activity reports on questionnaires are notoriously inaccurate and it is very difficult to establish how fit someone really is based on their answers to a questionnaire.

It is far better to measure fitness directly. This can be done using a maximal treadmill exercise test [see the boxed text at the end of this endnote for more information on treadmill tests].

The study consisted of 10,224 men and 3,120 women who had received a complete preventive medical examination and had undertaken a maximal treadmill exercise test at the Cooper Clinic of the Institute for Aerobics Research. The participants were then followed for a little more than eight years for a total of 110,482 total person-years of observation.

The key results from this study are shown in Figure 4 on page 2399 and are explained, somewhat cryptically, in the paragraph starting with "The various analyses presented..." Basically, what the figure shows is the rates of death per 10,000 person-years for each level of maximum aerobic capacity for men and women as established with the treadmill tests. The white vertical boxes represent men and the shaded vertical boxes represent women.

Maximum aerobic capacity is measured in metabolic equivalents (METs) (see the boxed text for more information on METs). All-cause mortality rates decreased dramatically as maximum aerobic capacity increased. Less than 6 METs is very unfit and the decrease in mortality levels out at about 9 METs for women and 10 METs for men (scientists call the location where it levels out the asymptote). MET scores of 9 to 10 are levels of fitness that can be achieved without exercise

Maximal Treadmill Exercise Tests and METs

The standard way to measure fitness is to measure the amount of oxygen that your body is capable of using. This is usually referred to as VO2 max, which is the maximum amount of oxygen that the body can use in milliliters per kilogram of body weight per minute (ml/kg/min).

Basically, the more oxygen your body can use the bigger your aerobic engine. Think of it this way. A Ferrari is going to be able to go faster than a Honda Civic because it has a larger engine and can use more fuel per minute than the Civic can.

Your body is an aerobic engine and how much work you can do (how fit you are) is measured by how much oxygen you can consume. (By the way, hyperventilating – taking a lot of deep breaths quickly – isn't going to make you go faster any more than putting ten gallons of gas in a Civic's gas tank and only five gallons of gas in the Ferrari's gas tank is going to make the Honda go faster than the Ferrari.)

Originally, treadmill tests were designed to be used with a breathing apparatus that would capture how much oxygen was expelled by the person doing the test as the treadmill went faster and the rate of incline was increased. An example of a treadmill protocol is the Balke Test, a copy of which is found in Appendix 2. The person taking the test simply continues to walk until it gets to be too much and they decide to quit.

However, scientists quickly figured out that for any given treadmill protocol, VO2 max rates were very similar for each time duration. In other words, everyone who could keep going on the test for eight full minutes always came very close to a VO2 max of 26 and people who could keep going for fourteen minutes always came in with a VO2 max of around 37.

Therefore, they could dispense with the breathing apparatus and simply see how long anybody could stay with the test. The longer they stayed with the test, the bigger their fitness engine.

One of the nice things about VO2 max is that it is calibrated to each person's body. The biggest problem with using calories to measure energy expenditure is that the bigger you are the more energy is required for you to do certain kinds of tasks. For example, if you weigh 180 pounds and walk a mile you expend 100 calories.

If you weigh 210 pounds, you expend more calories walking that mile, and if you weigh 150 pounds, you expend fewer calories.

Because VO2 max is the amount of oxygen you use at any given time per kilogram of body weight, it automatically adjusts to your size.

To make things a little simpler, researchers often translate VO2 max into something called metabolic equivalents or METs. One MET equals a VO2 max of 3.5. Why 3.5? Because if you were sitting on the couch doing nothing and watching television your VO2 max is 3.5.

When you sit and watch television, you are expending one MET of energy. If you sit there for an hour, you've expended 1 MET hour of energy. If your VO2 max at the end of the treadmill test is 35, it is also 10 METs.

5. Myers,. J, Prakash M, Froelicher V, et al. "Exercise capacity and mortality among men referred for exercise testing." *N Engl J Med.* 2002;346:793– 801. (http://www.nejm.org/doi /pdf/10.1056/NEJMoa011858)

This study used data from the Veterans Administration health system. The database consisted of approximately 6,000 men who had been referred for a treadmill test for clinical reasons. Of these, 2,534 turned out not to have any clinical problems.

The study followed all the participants for about six years. Once again, the differences in all-cause mortality between those who were fit and those who were unfit were huge. The key graphic is Figure 2, found on page 798. The shaded vertical bars are for those subjects who did not have any clinical problems based on the treadmill test, and the white vertical bars are for those who had some type of cardiovascular disease.

The five sets of vertical bars are by quintile. What that means is that each group was divided in to five equal sections based on the results of the treadmill test. Since those with cardiovascular disease were as a group less fit than those who showed no symptoms, the highest quintile for that group starts at 10.7 METs, whereas the highest quintile for the non-symptomatic group starts at 13 METs.

As might be expected, those with cardiovascular disease had higher death rates than those without symptoms in every quintile except the least fit quintile. For the subjects without symptoms (normal subjects), the decline in all-cause mortality was most dramatic as they moved from the lowest quintile upward, with the effect beginning to level off at around 10 METs.

At about 10 METs, which is a level that can be achieved without exercise, the rate of all-cause mortality is approximately one third that of the least fit group. (You can achieve a fairly accurate estimate of the all-cause mortality rate at 10 METs by averaging the relative risk rates of the third and fourth quintile.)

6. Kokkinos P, Myers J, et al. "Exercise capacity and mortality in black and white men." *Circulation*. 2008;117:614–622. (http://circ.ahajournals.org/cgi/reprint/117/5/614)

   This study utilized the same Veterans Administration database used in the Myers study referenced above in Endnote 5. But because the study was published six years after the Myers study, the database had grown to over 15,000 participants. The group was followed for approximately seven and a half years.

   The key graphic is Figure 6, found on page 621. In this study the participants were divided into four groups (quartile) based on the level of fitness achieved. One of the key objectives of this study was to see if there were differences between African-American and Caucasian participants. Therefore, Figure 6 contains three sets of vertical bars showing all-cause mortality rates for each fitness quartile for the entire group of participants and for the two subsets.

   Once again, the reduction in all-cause mortality was enormous as fitness increased. At 10 METs, the rate of all-cause mortality is approximately one third that of the least fit group. (Here again you can make a reasonable guess as to the all-cause mortality rate at 10 METs by averaging the third and fourth quartile.)

Chapter 4: Drs. Morris, Blair, Wei, et al. Turn the World Upside Down—No One Notices

1. Paffenbarger RS Jr, Blair SN, Lee IM. "A history of physical activity, cardiovascular health and longevity: the

scientific contributions of Jeremy N Morris." *Int J Epidemiol.* 2001;30:1184–1192. (http://ije.oxfordjournals.org/content/30/5/1184.full.pdf+html)

See page 1187 in the left-hand column for a discussion of how Dr. Morris went about evaluating the impact of weight on the rate of heart disease.

2. Blair, S, Kohl, H, Paffenbarger, R, et al. "Physical Fitness and All-Cause Mortality, A Prospective Study of Healthy Men and Women." *JAMA* 1989; 262:2395–2401 (http://jama.ama-assn.org/content/262/17/2395.full.pdf+html)

This study was discussed at some length in Endnote 4 of the prior chapter. The key graphics relating to weight are found in Figure 2, which shows the results for the women in the study and Figure 3, which shows the results for the men. Figures 2 and 3 are found on page 2398 and 2399.

Each figure has six graphics. The one for weight is the bottom center one. Probably the thing that jumps out at you the most from these figures is just how dangerous it is to be seriously under weight (below BMI 20), especially if you are unfit. But for both men and women, the group of participants that were both the fittest and heaviest had the second lowest death rates of any of the nine groupings.

3. Barlow, C. E., Kohl, H.W. I., Gibbons, L.W., & Blair, S. N. (1995). "Physical fitness, mortality and obesity." *International Journal of Obesity and Related Metabolic Disorders*, 19, S44. Unfortunately, this study is not available online.

This study looked at over 25,389 men who were followed for an average of 8.5 years. All the men had a complete physical examination and undertook a treadmill test to determine their level of fitness.

The study is quite clever in its approach because it first looked at the all-cause mortality of the total population without regard to fitness. The results were much the same as in the Canadian study that we looked at in the endnotes for Chapter 3. As weight went down for the general population, so did all-cause mortality. The age adjusted rate of death per 10,000 man years for the BMI over 30 group was 41.2, for the BMI 27 to 30 group it was 33.5 and for the BMI under 27 group it was 29.6. (Table 2, page S42)

Then they looked at the same weight groups, but divided into five fitness subgroups (quintiles). The age-adjusted rates of death per 10,000 man years for the quintile that was least fit were BMI under 27–52.1; BMI 27 to 30–49.1; and BMI over 30–62.1.

For the two highest fitness quintiles (which were combined in the study), the age-adjusted rates of death per 10,000 man years were BMI under 27–20.0; BMI 27 to 30–19.7; and BMI over 30–18.0. (Table 3, page S42)

In other words, those who were fit had essentially the same age adjusted rates of death regardless of their weight. And even those who were fit in the heaviest BMI category had rates of death that were substantially below those in the low fit category at the lowest weight level (18.0 versus 52.1).

4. Lee, C. D., Jackson, A. S., & Blair, S. N. (1998). "U.S. weight guidelines: Is it also important to consider cardiorespiratory fitness?" *International Journal of Obesity*, 22, S1-S7. (http://www.ncbi.nlm.nih.gov/pubmed/9778090) (Abstract only)

5. Lee, C. D., Blair, S. N., & Jackson, A. S. (1999). "Cardiorespiratory fitness, body composition, and all-cause and cardiovascular disease mortality in men." *American Journal of Clinical Nutrition*, 69, 373–380. (http://www.ajcn.org/content/69/3/373.full.pdf+html)

Perhaps the biggest problem with BMI as a measurement tool is that it only looks at height and total weight. Since muscle is a bit heavier, someone who is quite strong and has a lot of muscle mass but not much fat tissue would show up having a very high BMI. Arnold Schwarzenegger would be classified as being way overweight.

The purpose of this study was to look directly at body composition. This was assessed by measuring waist circumference, by hydrostatic weighing (weighing people while they are immersed in a pool of water), and/or by skinfold thickness tests. All the participants had also taken a treadmill test to measure their maximum cardiovascular fitness levels.

All of the participants were then classified into six groups for body fatness and cardiorespiratory fitness level:

- Lean (less than 16.7 percent body fat)–fit and unfit
- Normal (16.7 to less than 25 percent body fat)–fit and unfit

- Obese (equal to or more than 25 percent body fat)–fit and unfit

The key data is summarized on page 375 in Table 2.

Among the three groups who were fit (lean, normal, and obese), the highest relative risk of death was for the lean group at 1.00 (this was used as the referent group). The lowest relative risk of death was for the fit, normal group at .80. In the middle was the group classified at obese with a relative risk of .93.

In each body fatness category, the all-cause mortality rate of those who were unfit was about double that of those who were fit. Lean was at 2.06, normal at 1.61 and obese at 1.92.

Clearly, fitness makes a huge difference in the rate of all-cause mortality regardless of weight and among the fit group, the difference in all-cause mortality rates between the normal and "obese" group was minimal.

6. Blair, S. N. & Brodney, S. (1999). "Effects of physical inactivity and obesity on morbidity and mortality: Current evidence and research issues." *Medicine and Science in Sports and Exercise*, 31, S646-S662. (http://www.ncbi.nlm.nih.gov /pubmed/10593541) (Abstract only)

This paper reviewed twenty-four studies that have examined the relationships between weight and fitness, and all-cause mortality, cardiovascular disease mortality, coronary heart disease, hypertension, type II diabetes, and cancer.

Although only the abstract is available for free online, the third sentence in the paragraph labeled "Results" says it all: "Summary results for all outcomes except cancer [due to insufficient data] were generally consistent in showing that active or fit women and men appeared to be protected against the hazards of overweight or obesity."

7. Wei, M., Kampert, J. B., Barlow, C. E., Nichaman, M. Z., Gibbons, L.W., Paffenbarger, R. S., Jr., & Blair, S. N. (1999). "Relationship between low cardiorespiratory fitness and mortality in normal-weight, overweight, and obese men." *Journal of the American Medical Association*, 282, 1547–1553. (http:// jama.ama-assn.org/content/282/16/1547.full.pdf+html)

Early on in the book when we were talking about research, I mentioned how researchers are often not the world's greatest communicators. And boy is that ever true with this article.

The key, earth-shaking, mind-blowing data that is depicted in the graphic in Chapter 4 comes from two lines of data in Table 2 on page 1550 of the study. Table 2 contains twenty-four lines of data and the key mind-blowing ones are the last two lines in the table.

Adiposity as Compared with...

I would be remiss if I did not mention one study that challenged all the prior work proving that fitness eliminated the health risks of carrying extra weight. The study is titled "Adiposity as Compared with Physical Activity in Predicting Mortality among Women." (Hu, F., Willett, W., Li, T., et al. *N Engl J Med* 2004;351:2694–703.) (http://www.nejm.org/doi/pdf/10.1056/NEJMoa042135)

The basic claim of the study is that fitness is a good idea, but you still have to lose weight in order to be healthy. The study used an existing database of about 116,000 nurses that had been established in 1976. Every two to four years, the nurses filled out extensive questionnaires regarding their moderate or vigorous physical activity. This was then correlated with the participants BMI levels and their death rates.

Now there's nothing wrong with using an existing database to do a study. People do it all the time. And while it is nowhere near as accurate as a treadmill test in determining fitness, using physical activity questionnaires, when applied to the general population, can give a reasonable approximation of the physical fitness of the participants. The study's authors were at pains to validate the questionnaires (see the physical activity paragraph on page 2695 of the study).

The key findings are reported in the "Death from Any Cause" section of Table 3 on page 2700. One quick look at this immediately tells you that something is very wrong with the study. Forget for a moment the issue of whether fitness eliminates the health risks of weight. Fifty years of research have conclusively demonstrated that individuals who are not fit at any weight level have at least double the risk of dying compared with people at the same weight who are fit.

However, as you look across the horizontal rows for the relative risk of death for each of the three BMI categories, you see a very different picture. In the under BMI 25 group, the risk of dying is only 55 percent higher for the unfit group.

It gets worse. For the 25 to 29.9 BMI group, the risk of dying is only 28 percent greater for the unfit group, and for the 30 and over BMI group, it is only 27 percent greater. Something is very wrong. It turns out that what is wrong is that this is a study of nurses. What's wrong with nurses? Nothing. It's what's right with nurses. Nurses as a group are highly fit. Nurses along with waiters, farm workers and many others are in professions classified as having High Occupational Activity. For nurses, their high levels of fitness derive primarily from the fact that they do a lot of walking.

In fact, a study in the nursing magazine *MedSurg* used pedometers to determine that nurses on a hospital floor will walk an average of 756 steps per hour, or a total of about 6,000 steps per eight hour shift. (Welton, J., Decker, M. et al. "How far do nurses walk?" *MedSurg Nursing*, Aug;15(4):213–6.) (http://findarticles.com /p/articles/mi_m0FSS/is_4_15/ai_n17214422/?tag=content;col1)

As we'll see in Chapter 7, that 6,000 steps, combined with the 4,000 steps that most people normally take day-to-day outside of work, provides a sufficient level of fitness to completely eliminate the health risks of carrying extra weight.

The problem is that the database used in the "Adiposity" study had no way of taking the occupational fitness resulting from walking into account (without issuing all the nurses pedometers, there would be no way that it could be taken into account).

Many nurses work in hospitals, others work in busy clinics or doctor's offices and also do a lot of walking. Others, however, have desk jobs and do a lot less walking on the job. But the study database did not use a treadmill test to determine fitness and relied only on a leisure time physical activity questionnaire that did not take into account the high occupational activity levels of nurses. As a result, you have many highly fit nurses who may not participate in much leisure time physical activity, but who are extremely fit, being classified by the study as unfit.

This fouls up the entire data set and makes it non-interpretable. The study simply does not tell us anything about the relationship among fitness, weight, and all-cause mortality.

The fifty years of research that prove that fitness cuts the risk of dying in half, and the twenty plus years of research that prove that fitness eliminates the health risks of carrying extra weight still stand.

Chapter 5: But How Can That Be?

1. Marlowe, F. "Hunter-Gatherers and Human Evolution." *Evolutionary Anthropology* 14:54 –67 (2005) (http://www.fas .harvard.edu/~hbe-lab/acrobatfiles/hg%20and%20human %20ev.pdf)

    This interesting study looks at many aspects of how human beings evolved as hunter gatherers. The estimate for how much hunter gatherers walk each day is found in Table 3 on page 63. Table 3 focuses on warm climate, non-equestrian foragers, which is the environment in which humans first evolved.

    In the "Traits" column in Table 3, go down to the next-to-last entry titled "Day range (km)." The study estimates that the daily range for women was 9.5 km, which equals 5.9 miles or 11,800 steps. For men, the estimate is 14.1 km, which is 8.7 miles or 17,400 steps.

Chapter 6: If the Answer is 10,000, the Question is...?

1. Dr. Kenneth Cooper, *Aerobics*, Bantam Books- Available used at Amazon

2. Dr. Kenneth Cooper, *The Aerobics Way*, Bantam Books- Available used at Amazon

3. *Harvard Men's Health Watch*, Vol 11, No. 10, May 2007 (page 2) (http://harvardpartnersinternational.staywellsolutionsonline .com/HealthNewsLetters/69,N0507a)

4. Manson, J. et al. "A prospective study of walking as compared with vigorous exercise in the prevention of coronary heart disease in women." *N Engl J Med* 1999; 341:650–658 (http:// www.nejm.org/doi/full/10.1056/NEJM199908263410904)

    What the study did was to take a large database of women (over 72,000) and look at their activity levels and rate of coronary events (basically heart attacks, both fatal and nonfatal) over a period of eight years. The key finding was that "The magnitudes of risk reduction associated with brisk walking and vigorous exercise are similar when total energy expenditures are similar." (P. 656–first paragraph in the right hand column)

And just to be sure, she did the whole study over again three years later with a different database of women (see next endnote).

5. Manson, J. et al. "Walking Compared with Vigorous Exercise for the Prevention of Cardiovascular Events in Women." *N Engl J Med* 2002; 347:716–725 (http://www.nejm.org/doi/pdf/10.1056/NEJMoa021067)

This study involved more than 73,000 women who were followed for approximately six years. The key finding was that "We observed similar magnitudes of risk reduction with walking and vigorous exercise, and the results were similar among white women and black women as well as among women in different age groups and categories of body mass index." (Page 722–right-hand column)

6. Welton, J., Decker, M. et al. "How far do nurses walk?" *MedSurg Nursing*, Aug;15(4):213–6. (http://findarticles.com/p/articles/mi_m0FSS/is_4_15/ai_n17214422/?tag=content;col1)

This is the same study that we referenced in the "adiposity" box in the endnotes for Chapter 4. The exact number of steps that they found that nurses on a hospital floor took was an average of 756 per hour.

7. The original article is available only in abstract online. However, Dr. Paffenbarger wrote an excellent book called *LifeFit* that provides a very readable overview of the results of his research. See especially Chapter 2 and the chart on page 25.

8. Ohta T, Kawamura T, Hatano K., et al. "Effects of exercise on coronary risk factors in obese middle aged subjects." *Jpn Circ J.* 1990 Nov;54(11):1459–64. (http://www.researchgate.net/publication/20869134_Effects_of_exercise_on_coronary_risk_factors_in_obese_middle-aged_subjects) (Abstract only)

This study had a number of objectives, but one of the things it did was to measure the cardiovascular fitness of twenty-five participants in the program. After they got the group up to 10,000 steps, they asked them to take a partial treadmill test. Their average VO2 at that point was 25.4 ± 3.8. But that was not their maximum aerobic capacity.

That was because the researchers were being perhaps a bit overly cautious and terminated the tests when the participants reached 80 percent of their theoretical maximum heart rate (which is calculated by taking the number 220 and subtracting the person's age). Since the average age of the participants was approximately fifty years old, their predicted maximum heart rate would be 170 beats per minute. 80 percent of that would be 136. This is far less than the average person can achieve. In fact, in some studies people that don't at least achieve 85 percent of their predicted maximum heart rate are excluded on the grounds that this is probably an indication that they have some other underlying disease condition.

Fortunately, there is a lot of good data available to let us extrapolate from 80 percent of maximum heart rate to maximum exertion. For example, in Froelicher, V., Thompson A. "Prediction of maximal oxygen consumption–comparison of the Bruce and Balke treadmill protocols." *Chest* 1975;68;331–336 (http://chestjournal.chestpubs.org/content/68/3/331.full.pdf) [7a], on page 334 in Table 4, we can see that under the Bruce protocol, at the six minute mark, the participants had a heart rate of 133 and oxygen consumption of 24.3 ± 3.0. This is almost exactly the parameters of the Ohta study at 80 percent of maximal heart rate.

The same group at the ninth minute had a heart rate of 164 and oxygen consumption of 35.9 ± 4.2. 164 is sufficiently below the average maximal heart rate of the participants in the Ohta that we can assume that most or all of them could have reached this level had they been permitted to and thus their oxygen consumption should have been in the same range. And oxygen consumption of 35.9 ± 4.2 is the equivalent of 10.3 METs ± 1.2 METs.

Thus, we can be reasonably sure that someone who walks 10,000 steps will have a maximum aerobic capacity of between 9 and 10.5 METs.

9. Interview with Andrea Dunn by Peter Jaret of Consumer Health Interactive. (http://www.cvshealthresources.com/topic/exliteqa)

10. Tudor-Locke C, Bassett DR Jr. "How many steps/day are enough? Preliminary pedometer indices for public health." *Sports Med.* 2004;34(1):1–8. (http://www.ncbi.nlm.nih.gov/pubmed/14715035) [Abstract only]

11. Tudor-Locke C, Bassett DR Jr. "BMI referenced cut points for pedometer-determined steps per day in adults." *J Phys Act Health.* 2008;5 Suppl 1:S126–39. (http://www.aacorn .org/uploads/files/BMIReferencedCutPointsforPedometer DeterminedStepsperDayinAdults.pdf)

The quote is found on page 137 in the paragraph starting with "In 2004..."

12. Interview with David Bassett by Carol Krucoff, December 6, 1999

13. Here are a couple of examples:

13a. Thompson, D. L., J. Rakow, and S. M. Perdue. "Relationship between Accumulated Walking and Body Composition in Middle-Aged Women." *Med. Sci. Sports Exerc.*, Vol. 36, No. 5, pp. 911–914, 2004. (http://journals.lww.com/acsm-msse /Abstract/2004/05000/Relationship_between_Accumulated_ Walking_and_Body.26.aspx) (Abstract Only)

This study recruited eighty women aged forty to sixty-six to see if their habitual step counts were in any way correlated to their weight. Weights ranged from BMI 18.3 to BMI 53.3. Step counts ranged from 3,407 to 16,729. (Table 1, page 912)

The study found that there was a clear correlation. Participants walking fewer than 6,000 steps a day had average BMI of 29.3. Participants walking 6,000 to 9,999 steps per day had average BMI of 25.6. Participants who exceeded 10,000 steps a day had an average BMI of 23.6. (Table 3 and Figure 1, page 913)

13b. Dwyer, T. et al., "Association of change in daily step count over five years with insulin sensitivity and adiposity: population based cohort study." *BMJ* 2011; 342:c7249 (http:// www.bmj.com/content/342/bmj.c7249.full)

The objective of this study was to measure the impact of step count on insulin sensitivity. Type II diabetes is essentially the result of declining insulin sensitivity wherein the signaling mechanism of insulin is reduced and thus cells within the body cannot absorb sufficient glucose.

The study concludes on page 7 that a person who was sedentary at the start of the program, but who was able to build up to 10,000 steps each day "would have a threefold improvement in HOMA insulin sensitivity compared with a similar person who increased his or her steps" by only 3,000 steps a day, five days a week.

Chapter 7: It's All about How I Look, Stupid

1. *Health At Every Size: The Surprising Truth About Your Weight,* Linda Bacon, PhD, BenBella Books 2010

   The first part of this book describes in a very clear and readable way how the body reacts to attempts to lose weight and its mechanisms to protect itself against weight loss. It also describes some of the political aspects of the Obesity Epidemic, something that we will look at in more detail shortly.

   The second part of the book describes the Health At Every Size concept and process in great detail. The book also has an excellent resources section in the back.

2. Some places to start would include:
   - The Association for Size Diversity in Health (http://www.sizediversityandhealth.org/index.asp)
   - Healthy Weight Network (http://www.healthyweight.net/)
   - Body Image Health (http://www.bodyimagehealth.org/)
   - Body Positive (http://www.bodypositive.com/)

3. Bacon L, Stern JS, et al., "Size acceptance and intuitive eating improve health for obese, female chronic dieters." *J Am Diet Assoc.* 2005 Jun;105(6):929–36. (http://fog.ccsf.edu/lbacon/documents/JADAHAESstudy2005_105.pdf)

   This study is largely written in normal English and is worth reading in its entirety to get a sense of the really positive impact that the HAES program had on the participants.

4. Provencher V, Bégin C., et al. "Short-term effects of a "health-at-every-size" approach on eating behaviors and appetite ratings." *Obesity* (Silver Spring). 2007 Apr;15(4):957–66. (http://www.nature.com/oby/journal/v15/n4/pdf/oby2007113a.pdf)

   The investigators in the study divided 144 participants into three groups—a HAES group, a social support group, and a control group. The researchers concluded (on page 965) that "a HAES approach could have beneficial effects of particular eating behaviors and appetite sensations, when compared with the social support intervention or a control group."

5. Provencher V, Bégin C., et al., "Health-At-Every-Size and eating behaviors: 1-year follow-up results of a size acceptance intervention." *J Am Diet Assoc.* 2009 Nov;109(11):1854–61. (http://www.ncbi.nlm.nih.gov/pubmed/19857626) (Abstract only)

This study was a follow-up to the study referenced above in Endnote 4. The study found that over the longer term, the HAES program had beneficial effects as compared to the social support or the control groups.

Chapter 8: I Still Want to Take It Off, I Want to Take It All Off

1. Caroline R. Richardson, MD, et al. "A Meta-Analysis of Pedometer-Based Walking Interventions and Weight Loss." *Annals of Family Medicine* 6:69–77 (2008) (http://www.annfammed.org/cgi/reprint/6/1/69)

The detailed results from the nine studies reviewed by this paper are found in Table 2 on page 72. It shows the step count pre-intervention and post-intervention and weight levels pre-intervention and post-intervention. The final column shows weight changes in kilograms.

The paper concludes on page 74 in the first paragraph that "The average participant in a pedometer-based walking program without dietary change can expect to lose a modest amount of weight on the order of 1 kg."

2. *Health At Every Size: The Surprising Truth About Your Weight,* Linda Bacon, PhD, BenBella Books 2010

See Chapter 1 for a very complete, non-technical explanation of the entire set point process.

Chapter 9: Dieting and Fitness, Perfect Together?

1. Pavlou KN, Krey S., "Exercise as an adjunct to weight loss and maintenance in moderately obese subjects." *Am J Clin Nutr* 1989 49: 5 1115S-1123S (http://www.ajcn.org/content/49/5/1115.full.pdf)

We will talk a lot more about this study shortly. Look at Figure 6 on page 1122. There you will see that during the eight-week treatment period (that is the time that they went on a starvation diet), the fitness group, represented by the solid line, lost a bit more weight than the non-fitness group, represented by the dashed line.

Chapter 11: I Don't Eat That Much—Why Can't I Keep the %#&*^# Weight Off?

1. "The Truth about Dieting." *Consumer Reports*, June 2002, Vol. 67, Issue No.6.

The best way to access this online is probably through your local library. Most will have the EBSCO system available for library members. Usually you can access it through the library's online system and then just enter your library card or some other ID that your librarian will explain to you.

Chapter 12: Keeping It Off

1. Pavlou KN, Krey S., "Exercise as an adjunct to weight loss and maintenance in moderately obese subjects." *Am J Clin Nutr* 1989 49: 5 1115S-1123S (http://www.ajcn.org /content/49/5/1115.full.pdf)

The key graphic in this study is Figure 6, which can be found on page 1122. This graphic is a bit convoluted. I guess they were trying to save space by graphing all of the different groups together in one graphic. However, if you follow each of the lines carefully, you can see the various lazy "V," reclining "L," or lazy "U" shapes.

Also, at first glance, the graphic doesn't appear to exactly fit the lazy "V," reclining "L," or lazy "U" shapes that we described in Chapter 13. That is because of the way the bottom scale is set up. The left half of the bottom scale is eight weeks and the right half of the bottom scale is seventy-eight weeks. Thus, in reality the upward slopes on the right hand are much flatter (more "lazy") than they appear.

The fitness program for the fitness groups equaled the expenditure of approximately 1,500 calories per week. This is also described in Item 4 at the bottom of the left-hand column on page 1122.

Note that it is referred to as 1,500 kcal per week. That is because, technically speaking, a calorie is the amount of energy required to increase the temperature of 1 gram of water

1°C. What we call a calorie is technically a kilo calorie. It is the amount of energy required to raise the temperature of 1 kg of water 1°C. Therefore, in the scientific literature you'll often see kcal used in the notation.

2. Jakicic JM, Marcus BH, "Effect of exercise on 24-month weight loss maintenance in overweight women." *Arch Intern Med.* 2008 Oct 27;168(19):2162. (http://archinte.ama-assn .org/cgi/reprint/168/14/1550.pdf)

The key chart in this study is Figure 4 located on page 1556. Here the chart looks much more like our lazy "V" and reclining "L" because the horizontal scale is even all the way across. In this study weight loss maintenance occurred for the group expending at least 2,000 kcal week in the fitness program.

As you'll see as we go through a few more of these studies, the required energy expenditure levels range between about 1,500 kcal per week to about 2,400 kcal per week. Clearly, this is the right zone, but it can be able frustrating when you're trying to figure out exactly what level of energy you need to expand in order to maintain weight loss. We will discuss this in more detail in Chapter 13.

3. Fogelholm M., Kukkonen-Harjula K., "Does physical activity prevent weight gain—a systematic review." *Obes Rev.* 2000 Oct;1(2):95–111. (http://www.ncbi.nlm.nih.gov /pubmed/12119991) (Abstract only)

This study reviewed a number of papers that have examined the issue of physical activity and weight regain. Their conclusion was that an increase in physical activity in the range of 1,500 to 2,000 kcal per week was associated with improved weight maintenance.

4. Donnelly, J., Blair, S. et al. "Appropriate physical activity intervention strategies for weight loss and prevention of weight regain for adults." *Med Sci Sports Exerc.* 2009 Feb;41(2):459–71. (http://www.ncbi.nlm.nih.gov/pubmed/19127177) (Abstract Only)

This paper was also a review of the literature. One section focused on weight regain. Despite some grumps and harrumphs about studies not using enough randomization, the study concluded that the expenditure of an additional 300 calories per day in walking activities is "likely to be associated" with weight maintenance.

300 calories per day is equivalent of 6,000 steps, and since we assume the average person takes 4,000 steps a day prior to initiating any fitness activities, an extra 300 calories per day equals a 10,000 step per day fitness program.

Chapter 13: 10,000 Does It Again

1. Min, L., Djousse, L., "Physical Activity and Weight Gain Prevention." *JAMA*. 2010;303(12):1173–1179 (http://jama .ama-assn.org/content/303/12/1173.full.pdf+html)

   The key conclusion can be found at the bottom of column one and the top of column 2 on page 1177. They identified 4,540 women (13.3 percent of the study) who had a BMI of 25 at the start of the study and gained less than 2.3 kg (5 pounds) during the study period, which was twelve years. That group's mean activity level was 21.5 MET hours per week.

2. *The LA Times*, March 24, 2010 (http://articles.latimes.com/2010 /mar/24/science/la-sci-women-weight-gain24-2010mar24)

3. *The Cleveland Leader*, March 24, 2010 (http://www .clevelandleader.com/node/13435)

4. *Bloomberg Businessweek*, March 23, 2010 (http://www .bloomberg.com/apps/news?pid=email_en&sid=a9nNSVFs6E90)

Chapter 14: Getting to 10,000

1. Rails-To -Trails—Google Maps (http://maps.google .com/maps?hq=http://maps.google.com/help/maps /directions/biking/mapplet.kml&ie=UTF8&ll=37.687624, -122.319717&spn=0.346132,0.727158&z=11&lci=bike &dirflg=b&f=d&utm_campaign=en&utm_medium=ha&utm_ source=en-ha-na-us-sk-bd&utm_term=biking%20 directions)

Chapter 19: Committing Hari Kari— Non-Fatal (Mostly) Version

1. Wikipedia has a good description of these procedures and some not too graphic diagrams. (http://en.wikipedia.org /wiki/Bariatric_surgery)

2. Marketdata Enterprises is a large market research company with particular expertise in obtaining market research for the diet industry. If you are curious to get a glimpse as to how this industry thinks, a visit to their website (http://www.marketdataenterprises.com/DietMarket.htm) is definitely worthwhile. Their subsidiary site, Diet Busine$$Watch (http://www.dietbusinesswatch.com/Home_Page.html), provides lots of good, up-to-the-minute breaking news on the diet industry. As you can see from their name/logo (yes those dollar signs are part of the logo) this industry is all about the money.

3. Go down to the fifth bullet point under major findings. (http://www.emaxhealth.com/69/11203.html)

4. Flum DR, Dellinger EP. "Impact of gastric bypass operation on survival: a population-based analysis." *J Am Coll Surg.* 2004 Oct;199(4):543–51. (http://www.permanente.net/homepage/kaiser/pdf/32640.pdf)

The study examined 3,328 patients who had had a bariatric procedure. They found that 1.02 percent of the patients died while in the hospital and that another .88 percent of patients died within thirty days of their procedure for a total thirty day mortality of 1.9 percent (see the last paragraph on page 545). They also found that the death rates within thirty days of hospital discharge for inexperienced surgeons who had performed nineteen or fewer procedures was 4.7 times higher than for surgeons who were more experienced (first paragraph on page 546).

5. Encinosa WE, Bernard DM, et al. "Healthcare utilization and outcomes after bariatric surgery." *Med Care.* 2006 Aug;44(8):706–12. (http://www.ncbi.nlm.nih.gov/pubmed/16862031) (Abstract only)

6. Himpens J, Cadière GB, Bazi M, Vouche M, Cadière B., Dapri G. "Long-term Outcomes of Laparoscopic Adjustable Gastric Banding." *Arch Surg.* 2011 Mar 21. (http://www.ncbi.nlm.nih.gov/pubmed/21422330) (Abstract only)

7. As quoted in *SELF Magazine*: "The Miracle Weight Loss that isn't." Aug. 2008 (http://www.self.com/health/2008/07/risks-of-gastric-bypass-surgery?currentPage=1)

8. http://obesitysurgery-info.com

9. Flum DR, Dellinger EP. "Impact of gastric bypass operation on survival: a population-based analysis." *J Am Coll Surg.* 2004 Oct;199(4):543–51. (http://www.permanente.net/homepage/kaiser/pdf/32640.pdf)

   The study found that "Once surgical patients survived to the first year, the risk of dying during follow-up was 33 percent lower than non-operated, morbidly obese patients" (first paragraph under "Discussion" on page 547).

10. Adams TD, Gress RE, Smith SC, et al. "Long-term mortality after gastric bypass surgery." *N Engl J Med.* 2007 Aug 23;357(8):753–61. (http://www.nejm.org/doi/pdf/10.1056/NEJMoa066603)

    The design of the study was actually quite interesting. They took about 10,000 patients who had undergone gastric bypass surgery and about 10,000 very heavy persons who had applied for driver's licenses. Since the driver's license application required a person to indicate their height and weight, they were able to closely match 7,925 surgical patients with a similar number of control subjects with whom they were matched for age, sex and body mass index. However, they had no way to match them for health status or co-morbidities. They then followed these two groups for approximately seven years and were able to determine rates of death for each group using the National Death Index.

    Their key finding is in the first line of Table 2 on page 757. In the column labeled "Matched Subjects," the control group experienced 57.1 deaths per 10,000 person years versus 37.6 deaths per 10,000 person years for the surgery group which translates to an all-cause mortality reduction of 34 percent.

11. Matthew L. Maciejewski, PhD; Edward H. Livingston, MD; et al., JAMA. Published online June 12, 2011. doi: 10.1001/jama.2011.817, Survival Among High-Risk Patients After Bariatric Surgery (http://jama.ama-assn.org/content/early/2011/06/07/jama.2011.817.full.pdf+html)

    The problem with conducting these kinds of studies is that you cannot do a prospective (before the fact) randomized trial.

Imagine trying to get 500 people together who were considering bariatric surgery, arbitrarily dividing them into two groups of 250 each, and then assigning one group to go into surgery and the other not to have the surgery. That simply could not be done. As a result, these studies have to be retrospective (after the fact). What the researchers have to do is try to match the characteristics of those who underwent surgery with a similar group of people who did not.

The enormous advantage of this study was that all the 850 surgical patients involved were part of the Veterans Administration health system. The researchers were able to access a massive database of more than 41,000 Veterans Administration patients in order to develop extremely close matches for each of the 850 surgical patients and were able to include health status and co-morbidities as part of the matching criteria. Thus, the comparisons were far more accurate than was possible for the studies mentioned in the previous two endnotes.

12. Bloomberg news article, December 3, 2010 (http://www.bloomberg.com/news/2010-12-03/allergan-wins-fda-panel-s-backing-to-use-obesity-device-for-more-patients.html)

Chapter 20: Weight Loss Drugs—Forcing a Healthy System to Malfunction

1. Thomas A. Wadden PhD (Editor), Albert J. Stunkard MD (Editor), *Handbook of Obesity Treatment*, The Guilford Press 2004 (http://www.amazon.com/dp/1593850948)

   Chapter 15 of this book, written by George A. Bray (page 317), provides a very thorough review of the history of obesity drug treatment disasters.

2. Wikipedia entry for Orlistat (http://en.wikipedia.org/wiki/Orlistat)

   The FDA website details its current investigation. (http://www.fda.gov/Drugs/DrugSafety/PostmarketDrugSafety InformationforPatientsandProviders/DrugSafety InformationforHeathcareProfessionals/ucm179166.htm)

3. Matthew A. Weir, MD; Michael M. Beyea, PhD; et al. "Orlistat and Acute Kidney Injury: An Analysis of 953

Patients." *Arch Intern Med.* 2011;171(7):703–704. doi:10.1001/archinternmed.2011.103

The researchers looked at the case records of 953 people using Orlistat. They found that in the year prior to starting to use the drug, one-half of 1 percent of the new users were hospitalized for kidney problems. During the next year, the number of hospitalizations for kidney problems jumped to 2 percent, or a 300 percent increase.

This study is not available online and it does not have an abstract. A brief overview of the study can be found at: (http://www.urologytoday.net/article/roches-diet-drug-tied-to-kidney-damage/)

4. Davidson MH, Hauptman J, DiGirolamo M, "Weight control and risk factor reduction in obese subjects treated for 2 years with Orlistat: a randomized controlled trial." *JAMA.* 1999 Jan 20;281(3):235–42. (http://jama.ama-assn.org/content/281/3/235.full.pdf+html)

This study was funded by Hoffman-La Roche, the pharmaceutical company that markets the prescription version of Orlistat. Obviously, it will present the best possible case for the drug. It started out with well over 800 participants and ended up two years later with under 400 participants left (exactly how do you lose half of your study population in just 24 months?)

In any case, Figure 2 on page 239 shows the weight loss and regain for patients taking two different doses of Orlistat, a placebo group and a group that used Orlistat for the weight loss period, and then a placebo during the weight regain period.

5. A more comprehensive review can be found at a website called DrugLib.com. (http://www.druglib.com/druginfo/xenical/description_pharmacology/)

Of particular interest is their review of a study that followed 3,000 participants for a more realistic period of four years. Figure 1, about three quarters of the way down the webpage, shows the same pattern of weight regain for the patients on Orlistat.

Chapter 21: Weight Loss Programs

1. Tsai AG, Wadden TA. "Systematic review: an evaluation of major commercial weight loss programs in the United States." *Ann Intern Med.* 2005 Jan 4;142(1):56–66. (http://www.annals.org/content/142/1/56.abstract) (Abstract only)

2. Grodstein F, Levine R, Troy L, "Three-year follow-up of participants in a commercial weight loss program. Can you keep it off?" *Arch Intern Med.* 1996 Jun 24;156(12):1302–6. (http://archinte.ama-assn.org/cgi/content/abstract/156/12/1302) (Abstract only)

   An editorial in the same issue discussing the article and confirming its conclusions is available in full. (http://www.ajcn.org/content/88/5/1185.full.pdf)

Chapter 23: The Magic, Glowing Amberonium-Zircrohmic Weight Loss Pentagon

1. YouTube video showing Antonio Krastev setting a world record of 475 pounds in the snatch competition (http://www.youtube.com/watch?v=hD3WP6xQW4Y)

2. Recall of Joyful Slim Herb Supplement (http://www.fda.gov/Safety/Recalls/ucm219962.htm)

3. Tang MH, Chen SP, et al., "Case series on a diversity of illicit weight-reducing agents: from the well known to the unexpected." *Br J Clin Pharmacol.* 2011 Feb;71(2):250–3. (http://onlinelibrary.wiley.com/doi/10.1111/j.1365-2125.2010.03822.x/pdf)

   The authors of the study obtained eighty-one over-the-counter "slimming products" from 66 patients with poisoning symptoms. The products were subjected to laboratory analysis to determine their contents. Table 1 on page 251 shows the prevalence of the various illicit agents detected in the products.

   Worse yet, many of the products had multiple illicit agents as shown in Table 2 on page 252.

4. "There's 'nothing but danger associated with' cleansing. 'It is a practice to be condemned.'" Dr. Michael Gershon, Chairman

of Columbia University's Department of Anatomy and Cell Biology as quoted in *Bloomberg Businessweek*, February 27, 2011 pp. 77–79. (http://www.businessweek.com/magazine /content/11_09/b4217077879973.htm)

Chapter 24: The Obesity Reseachaganda Machine Just Keeps Going, and Going and Going

1. Obesity Care May Cost Twice Previous Estimates. (http://www.msnbc.msn.com/id/39693316/ns /health-diet_and_nutrition/)

2. Nearly 30 percent of Americans Likely to Have Diabetes by 2050 (http://www.articlesbase.com/science-articles/nearly-30 -of-americans-likely-to-have-diabetes-by-2050–3528870 .html)

3. UnitedHealth Predicts $3.4 Trillion Diabetes Decade (http:// www.bloomberg.com/news/2010–11–23/unitedhealth-says -diabetes-will-cost-3-4-trillion-over-the-next-decade.html)

4. Life Expectancy for Today's Youth Cut Short by Obesity (http://www.medicalnewstoday.com/articles/213559.php)

5. Cost of Obesity Approaching $300 Billion a Year (http://www. usatoday.com/yourlife/health/medical/2011–01–12-obesity -costs-300-bilion_N.htm)

6. Obesity Weighs down Cities' Budgets. Trimming Obesity Would Save U.S. Cities Millions in Healthcare Costs, Study Finds (http://www.webmd.com/fitness-exercise /news/20110127/obesity-rates-weigh-down-cities-budgets)

7. Why Are Men Getting So Tubby? (http://news.ebonybay.com /health/27322-Why-are-men-getting-tubby.html)

8. Bariatric Surgery Cuts Pounds, and Adds Years (http://www .msnbc.msn.com/id/41357739/ns/health-diet_and_nutrition/)

9. Study: Being Even a Little Fat a Health Risk (http://www .cbsnews.com/stories/2010/12/02/health/main7109429 .shtml)

10. Global Obesity Rates Are Doubling: New Worldwide Study (http://www.examiner.com/metabolic-syndrome-in-national /global-obesity-rates-are-doubling-new-worldwide-study)

Chapter 25: Celebrating "Obesity Epidemic" Day

1. Mokdad AH, Marks JS, Stroup DF, Gerberding JL, "Actual causes of death in the United States, 2000." *JAMA.* 2004 Mar 10;291(10):1238–45. (http://jama.ama-assn.org /content/291/10/1238.abstract) (Abstract only)

   This article claimed that obesity was the second-leading cause of death in the US after tobacco. In the abstract, you will see in the paragraph labeled "Results," and that 400,000 deaths are attributable to "poor diet and physical inactivity." However when you get into the article, what you discover is that "to assess the impact of poor diet and physical inactivity on mortality, we computed annual deaths due to overweight." And later on in the article they state that "overweight would account for the major impact of poor diet and physical inactivity on mortality." In other words, all those 400,000 deaths were actually attributable to obesity.

   However, when you try to follow their logic or their statistical methodology it gets very confusing very quickly, and as we'll discuss in Chapter 26, it turns out that there was a very good reason for that, namely that the whole thing was a complete manipulation job..

2. Glenn A. Gaesser, *Big Fat Lies: The Truth About Your Weight and Your Health*, Gurze Books, 2002; especially Chapters 1 and 2.

3. Waaler HT. "Height, weight and mortality. The Norwegian experience." *Acta Med Scand Suppl.* 1984;679:1–56. Not available online.

   This study, covering more than 1.7 million Norwegians, was one of the largest epidemiological studies ever conducted. It found that the longest life expectancy was BMI 21–27 for men and BMI 23–27 for women. (Figures 15 and 16 on page 23) That's exactly right. The so-called overweight folks, those with a BMI of 26 or 27 had the same life expectancy as those in the so-called normal BMI under 25 group.

   At the time, nobody was considering dividing the population into fit and unfit groups which obviously is what is needed to get a true reading on the situation. However, this was the type of information that was available and was, of course, ignored.

4. J. Eric Oliver, *Fat Politics: The Real Story behind America's Obesity Epidemic*, Oxford University Press, USA; 1 edition (September 14, 2006) p. 29 and footnote 40.

5. Linda Bacon, PhD, *Health At Every Size: The Surprising Truth About Your Weight,* BenBella Books 2010 p. 152–153 and Footnote 373

6. Here are just a couple of the headlines:

   • **Obesity to Surpass Tobacco as Top U.S. Killer** (http://www.newscientist.com/article/dn4763-obesity-to-surpass-tobacco-as-top-us-killer.html)
   • **Government: Obesity, Inactivity Nearly as Deadly as Tobacco in us** (http://www.msnbc.msn.com/id/4486906/ns/health-fitness/)

Chapter 26—Something Is Very Rotten in Denmark

1. Linda Bacon, PhD, *Health At Every Size: The Surprising Truth About Your Weight,* BenBella Books 2010 p. 151

2. Eliot Marshall, "Public Enemy Number One: Tobacco or Obesity?" *Science* 7 May 2004: Vol. 304 No. 5672 p. 804 (http://www.sciencemag.org/content/304/5672/804.summary) (Abstract Only)

3. *Washington Times,* February 27, 2005 (http://www.washingtontimes.com/news/2005/feb/27/20050227-095255-6321r/print/)

4. A good summary of the entire set of events can be found at http://www.obesitymyths.com/myth2.2.htm.

Appendix 1A
Body Mass Index Chart
BMI 19–36

Body Weight (pounds)

Height	19	20	21	22	23	24	25	26	27	28	29	30	31	32	33	34	35	36
4' 10"	91	96	100	105	110	115	119	124	129	134	138	143	148	153	158	162	167	172
4' 11"	94	99	104	109	114	119	124	128	133	138	143	148	153	158	163	168	173	178
5'	97	102	107	112	118	123	128	133	138	143	148	153	158	163	168	174	179	184
5' 1"	100	106	111	116	122	127	132	137	143	148	153	158	164	169	174	180	185	190
5' 2"	104	109	115	120	126	131	136	142	147	153	158	164	169	175	180	186	191	196
5' 3"	107	113	118	124	130	135	141	146	152	158	163	169	175	180	186	191	197	203
5' 4"	110	116	122	128	134	140	145	151	157	163	169	174	180	186	192	197	204	209
5' 5"	114	120	126	132	138	144	150	156	162	168	174	180	186	192	198	204	210	216
5' 6"	118	124	130	136	142	148	155	161	167	173	179	186	192	198	204	210	216	223
5' 7"	121	127	134	140	146	153	159	166	172	178	185	191	198	204	211	217	223	230
5' 8"	125	131	138	144	151	158	164	171	177	184	190	197	203	210	216	223	230	236
5' 9"	128	135	142	149	155	162	169	176	182	189	196	203	209	216	223	230	236	243
5' 10"	132	139	146	153	160	167	174	181	188	195	202	209	216	222	229	236	243	250
5' 11"	136	143	150	157	165	172	179	186	193	200	208	215	222	229	236	243	250	257
6'	140	147	154	162	169	177	184	191	199	206	213	221	228	235	242	250	258	265
6' 1"	144	151	159	166	174	182	189	197	204	212	219	227	235	242	250	257	265	272
6' 2"	148	155	163	171	179	186	194	202	210	218	225	233	241	249	257	264	272	280
6' 3"	152	160	168	176	184	192	200	208	216	224	232	240	248	256	264	272	279	287
6' 4"	156	164	172	180	189	197	205	213	221	230	238	246	254	263	271	279	287	295
BMI	19	20	21	22	23	24	25	26	27	28	29	30	31	32	33	34	35	36

Body Weight (pounds)

Height	37	38	39	40	41	42	43	44	45	46	47	48	49	50	51	52	53	54
4'10"	177	181	186	191	196	201	205	210	215	220	224	229	234	239	244	248	253	258
4'11"	183	188	193	198	203	208	212	217	222	227	232	237	242	247	252	257	262	267
5'	189	194	199	204	209	215	220	225	230	235	240	245	250	255	261	266	271	276
5'1"	195	201	206	211	217	222	227	232	238	243	248	254	259	264	269	275	280	285
5'2"	202	207	213	218	224	229	235	240	246	251	256	262	267	273	278	284	289	295
5'3"	208	214	220	225	231	237	242	248	254	259	265	270	278	282	287	293	299	304
5'4"	215	221	228	234	240	246	250	256	262	267	273	279	285	291	296	302	308	314
5'5"	222	228	234	240	247	252	258	264	270	276	282	288	294	300	306	312	318	324
5'6"	229	235	241	247	253	260	266	272	278	284	291	297	303	309	315	322	328	334
5'7"	236	242	249	255	261	268	274	280	287	293	299	306	312	319	325	331	338	344
5'8"	243	249	256	262	269	276	282	289	295	302	308	315	322	328	335	341	348	354
5'9"	250	257	263	270	277	284	291	297	304	311	318	324	331	338	345	351	358	365
5'10"	257	264	271	278	285	292	299	306	313	320	327	334	341	348	355	362	369	376
5'11"	265	272	279	286	293	301	308	315	322	329	338	343	351	358	365	372	379	386
6'	272	279	287	294	302	309	316	324	331	338	346	353	361	368	375	383	390	397
6'1"	280	288	295	302	310	318	325	333	340	348	355	363	371	378	386	393	401	408
6'2"	287	295	303	311	319	326	334	342	350	358	365	373	381	389	396	404	412	420
6'3"	295	303	311	319	327	335	343	351	359	367	375	383	391	399	407	415	423	431
6'4"	304	312	320	328	336	344	353	361	369	377	385	394	402	410	418	426	435	443
BMI	37	38	39	40	41	42	43	44	45	46	47	48	49	50	51	52	53	54

Appendix 2A
Balke Treadmill Protocol for Women

Speed/Miles per Hour	% Grade	Minutes	METS
3.0	0	1	1.9
3.0	0	2	2.3
3.0	0	3	2.7
3.0	2.5	4	3.1
3.0	2.5	5	3.5
3.0	2.5	6	3.9
3.0	5	7	4.3
3.0	5	8	4.6
3.0	5	9	5.0
3.0	7.5	10	5.4
3.0	7.5	11	5.8
3.0	7.5	12	6.2
3.0	10	13	6.6
3.0	10	14	7.0
3.0	10	15	7.4
3.0	12.5	16	7.8
3.0	12.5	17	8.2
3.0	12.5	18	8.6
3.0	15	19	9.0
3.0	15	20	9.4
3.0	15	21	9.8
3.0	17.5	22	10.2
3.0	17.5	23	10.6
3.0	17.5	24	11.0
3.0	20	25	11.3
3.0	20	26	11.7
3.0	20	27	12.1
3.0	22.5	28	12.5
3.0	22.5	29	12.9
3.0	22.5	30	13.3

Appendix 2B
Balke Treadmill Protocol for Men

Speed/Miles per Hour	% Grade	Minutes	METS
3.3	0	1	4.7
3.3	2	2	5.1
3.3	3	3	5.5
3.3	4	4	5.9
3.3	5	5	6.3
3.3	6	6	6.8
3.3	7	7	7.2
3.3	8	8	7.6
3.3	9	9	8.0
3.3	10	10	8.4
3.3	11	11	8.8
3.3	12	12	9.2
3.3	13	13	9.6
3.3	14	14	10.0
3.3	15	15	10.5
3.3	16	16	10.9
3.3	17	17	11.3
3.3	18	18	11.7
3.3	19	19	12.1
3.3	20	20	12.5
3.3	21	21	12.9
3.3	22	22	13.3
3.3	23	23	13.7
3.3	24	24	14.2
3.3	25	25	14.6
3.3	26	26	15.0
3.3	27	27	15.4
3.3	28	28	15.8
3.3	29	29	16.2
3.3	30	30	16.6

Appendix 3
Working with Your Pedometer

A few more words about working with your pedometer, since it's going to be your constant companion. Pedometers can sometimes be temperamental little critters, and you need to make friends with them. Everyone's body type and walking style differs, and pedometers can also differ, so you need to take some time to ensure accuracy.

Count 50 or 100 steps while you're walking and compare that with your pedometer's count. Most pedometers will be quite accurate while you're walking steadily for some length of time. But some may be less accurate if you're doing a lot of walking back and forth around the house or at work. They can also sometimes be different if you are walking on a treadmill versus regular walking. Even the clothes you wear (different waistbands) can influence the count.

If a pedometer is very erratic or consistently more than 15 percent off, return it and buy another one. Otherwise, you may just need a period of checking your step count under different conditions to work out your personal profile. Let's say you manually count 100 steps about four times in one day and come up with pedometer counts of 82, 97, 92, and 88. This averages out at about 90, so you can add 10 percent to your grand total at the end of that day. Your count doesn't have to be perfect—you just need to be in the right general zone. Again, this is usually only necessary for your miscellaneous steps, not for when you go for a walk.

It might also be a good idea to try two or three pedometers for different kinds of walking, or in case you lose one or one breaks. They aren't that expensive, and they are worth their weight in gold.

Index

Who the Heck Is Mike Schatzki and Why Did He Write This Book?

Actually, I didn't have any intention of writing a book at all.

I'm a professional speaker. I go around the world giving speeches and I often conduct two day training programs helping people become better negotiators. And I thought, "I'm up on my feet for two days, I'm walking around during the class, so I must be fit."

As I got a bit older, I began to huff and puff a little bit as I climbed a flight of stairs and my energy level seemed a bit lower. But I'm a trainer, I'm in shape, I'm okay. You see, I had a black belt in denial.

But I wasn't the only one who was getting little a bit concerned. My wife Jeannie was also concerned about her fitness level, but she did something about it. She went out and took one of those fitness assessments. And then she started working out.

So you know, well, she's doing something about it, I better not just sit around, I'd better do something. So I figured, I'll take that fitness test and just ace it.

Do you know what they said? It was all lies! Slander, defamation of character! They said I was a middle-aged, out-of-shape, male. I'll sue!

The trouble was, they were being kind. The truth was that I was a terribly out-of-shape, middle-aged male. And you know, down deep, I really was a little concerned. Maybe I should do something about it. And so I started my journey to fitness.

Of course, at the time, I didn't know anything about 10,000 steps. Like everyone else, I assumed you had to exercise hard to get fit. And so I did. Sweat, get your heart rate up, no pain no gain. And of course, I made every mistake in the book.

There just had to be a better way. I started to do some research and it was just amazing how much the experts and researchers knew that the rest of us had no idea was out there. I figured, "I'm a professional speaker, I'll put together a speech and share all this new information with the world."

But when you give a speech, it's not just a matter of grabbing some facts and putting them into a nice verbal package. You have to have deep knowledge. You really need to know what you're talking about, not only to be sure that the information in the speech is accurate, but also so that you can answer questions from the audience during and after the program. That means serious research.

And so, over about a year's time, I accumulated a bunch of books and several hundred scientific research articles and put it all together in a speech. I christened myself "The Recovering Couch Potato" and started to present the speech, which I call "The No Sweat Couch Potato Recovery Program."

But research can have a sort of seductive quality about it, particularly if you're the kind of person who is easily intrigued by new information. As I read the research on fitness, I couldn't help bumping into discussions on weight and obesity and their relationship to fitness. And so inevitably, you follow the footnote trail. The paper you're reading mentions something interesting and there is a reference, so you go and get that article, and then there are couple of footnotes in that article, and you go on to the next and so on.

And so another bunch of books and a couple of hundred more research papers. And the more I read, the more amazed and appalled I became. Here was all this information that all these brilliant researchers had developed and that nobody was talking about. In fact, everybody was saying just the opposite.

Not okay. Time to set the record straight and speak truth to power.

And thus was born *The Great Fat Fraud*. I hope you enjoyed reading it and I hope that it will make a real difference in your life.

***

Mike Schatzki received his BA, Magna Cum Laude, Phi Beta Kappa, from Haverford College, and his MPA from Princeton University's Woodrow Wilson School of Public and International Affairs.

Mike lives in Northern New Jersey with his wife Jeanne and their cat Karma.

You can contact Mike via:
- Email—Mike@GreatFatFraud.com
- Facebook—www.facebook.com/greatfatfraud
- Twitter—@MikeSchatzki

13432752R00119

Made in the USA
Lexington, KY
10 February 2012